Also by Linda Ingalls

I May Be Crazy, But It's All Good

Praise for Where Do You Draw The Line?

"I want to thank you very much for your honesty and your comforting words, which were both bitter and sweet, all very much needed during a stressful time. I greatly appreciate you sharing your book, <u>Where do you draw the line?</u> with me. It contained so much 'critically' needed information that helped me to intelligently make some very difficult and emotional decisions. Your presence will be remembered like an angel, shining a little light into a very dark and difficult time." – Marcia Repaci

"Your book is so practical and informative. I appreciate it a lot." –Janine Whitaker

"Patients and their families have found this book to be an excellent source of comfort and education during the most trying of times...thumbs up...a must read." David Likosky, MD

"Through this book, I have witnessed many situations where without it, the patients and families would have been much more apprehensive to ask questions, discuss, and participate in their own care plan or the care for their loved one. It is a very valuable and heartfelt tool." – Kay Erickson, RN

Where do YOU draw the line?

An Insider's guide to effective Living Wills, Healing, and Critical care

By Linda Ingalls RN CCRN

2nd edition – published 2013 by CreateSpace
Previously published by Trafford Publishing in 2003

ISBN-13: 978-1490536903
ISBN-10: 1490536906
Library of Congress Control Number: 2013912753

Contact information:
Linda Ingalls: imlindai41@gmail.com
www.lindaingalls.com

This book is dedicated
to
Everyone who loves someone

Acknowledgements

To all of the people I have worked with, staff, patients and families thank you for all of the lessons you have taught me.

To my family and friends, thank you for your love and support throughout the years.

To Dane Kessler and Marta Grapensteter, RN thanks for your input.

To Love, thank you for guidance and correction. It's done! Now what?

Finally, to Lee, my husband and my friend, thanks for doing the original edit and encouraging me to do my best. Thanks for sharing your life with me. I love you this ∞ much.

———

Re-dedication to Lee:
He said "You told me I have the right to make my own choice."
And he did.
Be in peace, my love.
Leonidas Ingalls
1933 - 2003

TABLE OF CONTENTS

To YOU the Reader

I believe every adult should read this book, however, you do not have to read the *whole* book. Some of this information you may never need for yourself nor anyone you know. BUT, you do need to know the information in Part 1. Please read pages 15 -59 and 65 - 80.

The information in Part 2 can help make your life better in so many ways, and I highly recommend it.

Check out Part 3 when you need to know or are just curious.

PART ONE

THINGS TO KNOW

1

PURPOSE
(why I wrote this book)

I wrote this book for you and your loved ones.

In the USA, you are considered to be a Full Code i.e. we will automatically keep you alive no matter what, if we can, unless you tell us otherwise. Is this what you want? Is it what your loved ones want for you or for themselves? Have you all effectively communicated your healthcare wishes?

Hi, my name is Linda. I've been a nurse since 1975 and began critical care in 1981. One of the hardest things in my job is taking care of the unsuspecting patient or family who comes to the Critical Care Unit totally unprepared to make the major health care decisions that will be forced upon them. I want to inform and empower you to make decisions based upon Love not fear.

Making good decisions in a time of crisis is hard to do. It's worse if you've never thought about it. And how can you possibly make decisions for someone you love if you've never even talked about it? These situations should bring families together in love and support, but too often instead, there is indecision, arguing and guilt because nobody knows what their loved one would really want done. In that case, it's easy to feel out of control and victimized. But it doesn't have to be that way.

You need to understand what you are choosing to experience. There are some simple fundamental things you need to know to empower yourself and those you love. Understanding critical care issues will decrease fear, put life into perspective and promote peace of mind. Don't wait for a crisis. Knowing how to cope can help you survive critical care.

Knowledge is power. The purpose of this book is to give you information to help you make decisions, founded upon Love, that you can live with.

Part One has information and tips about resuscitation, life support, code status, palliative and comfort care, effective Living Wills, Power of Attorney for Healthcare, Physician Orders for Life Sustaining Treatment (POLST), and effective communication with doctors, etc.

Part Two focuses on coping and complimentary ways to create a healing environment.

Part Three discusses, in easy "lay-man language", some of the equipment and some of the common illnesses you may experience in critical care. You can browse this section, but please do read the introduction of Part Three - page 99 and the Ventilator section - page 132. *Remember, that technology, therapies, procedures and drugs will continue to evolve, but you can capture the basic concepts here and build on them as new treatment comes about.*

2

WHY BOTHER?
(why you need this information)

You may be wondering, *"Why the heck does she want me to think about this scary stuff. It's depressing, who wants to go there?"* Listen, I know that thinking about these things is scary and, believe me, nobody wants to think about it. BUT, it's way scarier to deal with things during a crisis, and then later have to live with results you may not have wanted. It's comfortable to be wrapped in a cocoon of ignorance and denial, thinking, "These things may happen, but not to me." But we will all be facing death in our lifetimes. Being in critical care can bring about major life changes, and most changes are hard to deal with--especially if you weren't expecting them.

My mortgage broker is fond of saying "You have to have an exit plan when you buy a home. I think it is empowering to have an "exit plan" for life, but, people are afraid that, *if they think about it*, they will cause it to happen. If you drive a car, do you carry a spare tire and a jack? Getting a flat tire isn't something you *dwell* upon. No. You just make your provisions and then get on with driving. Dying is a part of living. If you're prepared, you can plan for a "good death" the way you might plan for a "good birth", or a "good wedding." You don't dwell upon it. You just take care of business and then get on with the living! We don't always know when we're going to die, we just know we will. Our attitude toward death will determine whether or not we're victims. There's a great line from the book Tuesdays with Morrie. Morrie said, "When you know how to die, you know how to live." I believe that when you face dying you learn what's really important to you, change your priorities, and have a better life.

If you knew you had only one hour left to live, what would you regret not having done? What would you regret not having said? **Stop!** Think about this right now.

If you knew you were going to move to another country and would never see your family or your friends again, would you wait till the last minute to say everything you wanted to say? Would you regret not seeing or doing things you wanted to do? Or would you take the time before your move to say and do all that you could? Life is all about choosing. When you choose between two things you want, you pick the thing that is most important to you. In the end, whether or not you got to do everything you thought you wanted to do, you'll still have done all that is most important to you, and there'll be no regrets. It is a win/win situation.

And what of your parents, spouse, or adult children? If you're suddenly faced with the task of making major health care or life and death decisions for them, do you even have a clue as to what they'd want you to do? Would you know how to help them?

In the past, the medical system could only do so much to save your life. There wasn't much to think about because there were few choices, so public education didn't seem to be needed. Today, with transplants, better technology, and better drugs, we can do a whole lot more. And who knows where cloning and stem cell research will lead? You may have more options, but there are still many limitations.

In the old days when a person went on life support we were talking the end of the line. Today the question is *what kind* of life support do I need and for *how long*? In the past we thought only in terms of life and death, but now we must ask, "What will the *quality* of my life be? Will this treatment bring me back to the way I was, and if not, will it be a kind of life I would want?

In the past, doctors made these decisions. Today YOU and YOUR FAMILY make them.

If you want to have everything done for you or your loved one, we'll be there for you. But you need to understand what that means. You need to understand your options and what you're getting into. To make the best decisions you'll need information. So, where do you begin?

3

FUNCTION IS THE GUIDE
(how do you know what you want?)

First, let's just ask the big question: if your body is trying to die, do you want us to try to stop it or do you want us to allow you to have a peaceful death?

Of course, that answer will change as you live your life. So, if/when you do change your mind, make sure you communicate this. I will give you guidelines regarding communication later in this book.

Now let's say you want us to try to save your life. Great! Then we need to talk about what you want to achieve. Ask yourself what *level of disability* are you willing to live with? What is the *"basic level of functioning"* you need to make life worth living? *Where do you draw the line?* Here is a guideline I use with folks, starting with the most limiting disability and then going up in function:

1. **Is it okay to be in a coma?** One patient with cancer said that he wanted to keep going unless he was brain dead. Does that mean it was okay with him to live in a coma for the rest of his life? He said, "Yes." He was young with young children and was willing to live in a coma hoping that a cure could eventually be found.

2. **Is it important that you are conscious and can recognize loved ones?** Often when a person is in a "vegetative coma" they appear to be aware of people in the room and appear to respond even though medical wisdom says they are not. This can lead to a lot of

conflict in families on what to do. In my experience, if a person has, in the past, stated they would not want to be kept alive if they could not talk, eat, etc. then there is no conflict because a person in this condition will not be doing that.

3. **Is it important that you can communicate in some way?** This could be by blinking or raising your eyebrows; but, one patient said that she would need to be able to talk, to share her ideas, and give advice to help other people. It would be okay if she were paralyzed as long as she could talk. What she really wants is not to just talk; she wants to be able to think, to understand what someone is saying to her, and to be able to speak well enough that others would not consider it too great a task to listen to her.

4. **Is it important to you that you can eat food with your mouth?** Believe it or not, eating by mouth is very important to some people. They would rather not live if they cannot do this. For some people the danger in eating by mouth is that swallowing is an issue. They may choke and stop breathing; or, the food/liquid could be slowly going into the lungs which could cause a serious pneumonia and possibly a serious infection called Sepsis, and necessitate life support. So, my question is, if you want to eat, do you want to be put on life support if something goes wrong; or, do you want to eat and be a No Code? (see code status)

5. **Is it important that you can move your body in bed?**

6. **Is it important that you can get your body out of bed...with or without help?**

7. **Is it important that you can go to the bathroom by yourself?**

8. **Is it important that you can get around your home by yourself?**

9. **Is it important that you can take care of your home by yourself?**

10. **Is it important that you can get out of your home and take care of business by yourself?** Another lady said that if she could not be independent and take care of herself she wouldn't want to live. That allows for a lot of various disabilities including stroke, paraplegia, amputations, some brain damage, etc. Lots of people with disabilities live independent lives.

Another woman said any disability was unacceptable.

You get the picture? What do *you* need to make your life worthwhile?

Then, consider this: are you willing to do rehab for a month, a few months, a year, for as long as possible? Do you have an end point? How long are you willing to do rehab to get to that bottom line?

Knowing what you're willing to live with will be the guiding light for making health care decisions, including what kind of life support you want and how long you would want it. If you want it all, does that mean you're willing to live with any kind of loss of functioning? Think about it. While we may be able to keep you alive and even get you off of life support, there's no guarantee that you're going to like the life we've saved you for. Maybe you will, maybe you won't. This is why knowing your bottom line can be so helpful.

When you or your loved ones are making these decisions, take time to evaluate *why* you are making the choice you want. Be well informed about your options. That's the purpose of this book. If you're choosing to *not* have life support *for any reason* ask yourself why? If you're choosing this because life seems hopeless or because you feel like a burden to your family, you should talk to your family or seek counseling before making your decision. If you feel your family is pressuring you into making this decision, don't let them, get family counseling. End of life decisions are best made for spiritual and practical reasons.

On the other hand, if you want yourself or your loved one to have full life support for as long as possible, to "go down kicking and scratching", ask yourself why? We will all die someday. How sick does the mind or body have to be before it's okay to let go? One woman with severe Alzheimer's disease came to critical care because she was having irregular heartbeats. She lives at home with a 24-hour caregiver. Her son lives across the state and sees his mom for about an hour once a week. Her mind has deteriorated to the point where she can barely make a sound. She is fed through a tube. She lies in bed in a constant fetal position. It hurts her when we move her. Her hands are tied down because she pulls out her IV's. She's a Full Code. Although they've never discussed her wishes, her son insists everything be done to keep her alive. Do you think she would want us to do that? Would you want it if this were your loved one? Would you want this for yourself? You should know this answer.

4

DON'T FORGET THE MONEY

Now that you know what basic level of functioning you are willing to live with, you need to ensure you'll have the money for any care or equipment that you may need in both the acute care hospital and in long term care.

Maybe for you money isn't a consideration. Maybe you have a situation where you don't need to pay or can't pay and the government provides health care for you. To many of us, especially in the flux of healthcare reform, money is an important factor. The last time I checked a base cost for one day in a critical care unit was upward of $2000.

Some people are willing to spend whatever it takes to keep themselves or someone they love alive. How wonderful that they can do that! Some of my patients have told me they spent all of their savings, even sold their homes to pay for the care of their spouse and they were happy to do this. But, when the spouse died there was nothing left over to help take care of themselves. Most say they would not have done it differently, and some say it was among the happiest times of their life. But others, in hindsight, felt it would have been better for both them and their spouse to have lovingly let go and allowed a peaceful passing.

Most people do not know they even have a choice. For example one patient's doctor had sent her 100 miles from home to a university hospital for tests because she was dying, and he didn't know what to do. During our discussion about her wishes, she was shocked to learn that she had the right to refuse medical care. She was furious because she'd worked hard and saved her money to bequeath to her granddaughter for college. Now it was being used in an effort to prolong her own life. She was prepared for her death and not uncomfortable with the thought of dying. What made her happy was knowing she could do something great for her granddaughter.

Money should not be a factor in health care, but the reality is that money means a great deal. If you decide you can live with a major disability, who will take care of you? Who will provide for your financial support? Do you know what your insurance will pay for and what they won't pay for while you are in the hospital? Do you know what services it'll pay for when you leave the acute care hospital and need rehabilitation or long term hospitalization? Will it pay for in home care; or, custodial care? If so, for how long? What are the requirements for it to pay? Do you have a Supplemental insurance that is supposed to pay for these kinds of things? Read the fine print and make sure it covers what you want.

If you are looking at end of life care you still need to check out the financial costs for home, custodial or nursing care. You need to see whether or not you are eligible for Hospice care. You need to check out costs for funerals or cremations. In many states there are consumer oriented non-profit organizations that provide discounts on funeral and cremation services through mortuaries they have contracts with. You join with a low lifetime membership fee. These local organizations can be affiliated with others across the United States through the Funeral Consumers Alliance, thus allowing for services if you happen to die while traveling. In Washington State one fine organization is the People's Memorial Association. When you are dealing with end of life issues, there are many resources of help and information. One great place is: http://www.caringinfo.org.

Be sure to talk to people who know and understand the financial aspects of health care. Talk to insurance agents, financial planners, social workers, case managers, friends and family with experience. See if your local hospital has a "care network". This is a system of folks from a variety of specialties (like those I just mentioned) that help with information, filling out forms, planning your care, etc. They can steer you in the right direction and help you get where you need to be.

V

LIFE SUPPORT AND CODE STATUS

Now that you know where you want to draw the line and how much you're willing to pay for it, you need to have an idea of what you might have to go through. You need to know what life support is. Life support can be classed as Emergency, Critical, and Long Term. There are some distinct differences and a lot of overlap. This can be confusing to the patient or family trying to decide whether to start or stop life support. The bottom line is if you can't live without it, it's life support.

EMERGENCY LIFE SUPPORT (Resuscitation)

During an emergency, when you're either not breathing and/or your heart isn't beating in a way that'll allow your brain to get enough oxygen, you need ***basic life support*** - *CPR, cardiopulmonary resuscitation.* This is when someone is **pressing** on your chest to make the blood flow, and they're **breathing** for you with their mouth, or a mask, on your nose and mouth. Without this, you will die. If your heart is beating erratically, you'll also be getting electric shock if there is an *AED -automated external defibrillator* available. This is done to restore an effective heartbeat.

When the appropriate medical service is available, you may receive the life support of certain drugs. Most of these drugs are used to control your heartbeat: to kick-start it, to slow it down, or to speed it up.

You may also need a tube placed into your airway via your mouth or nose to help with your breathing. This is called *intubation*. Intubation and mechanical ventilation are discussed in detail in the Equipment section under LUNGS. I strongly urge you to read this section because this particular life support can be the most challenging one to experience, and it is the one where your coping ability can help you survive.

You may need more electric shocks for erratic, too fast, or too slow heart rhythms.

Sometimes you need drugs we call *pressors* to keep your blood pressure high enough to circulate blood to your brain and other organs. Some drugs help lower a critically high blood pressure. Other drugs help your heart muscle pump stronger.

If you need electric shocks, drugs, or intubation, this is called **advanced life support**. If you're in a situation where we are doing either basic or advanced life support, it's called a **CODE** situation.

CRITICAL CARE LIFE SUPPORT

If you've been "coded" you'll for sure have the breathing tube put in and eventually be connected to a ventilator, which is the life support machine for breathing. You will be brought to critical care.

But, you don't have to be in a code situation to need *critical care life support*. Don't misunderstand me, not all patients who come to critical care need life support. People come into the critical care unit for many reasons: a sudden severe illness like a heart attack, bad pneumonia, an accident, bleeding ulcer, stroke, infection, major surgery, etc.

However, no matter *why* you came to critical care, *if* at any time, you start having trouble with ventilation -- by that I mean you have trouble getting enough oxygen into your body; trouble getting carbon dioxide out of your body; or you're too weak to cough the spit out of your lungs – you will be intubated and connected to a ventilator. This is a big part of critical care life support. Being intubated is probably the most uncomfortable and challenging life support you'll experience. You must perceive it as your friend while you're in need. See it as your personal tool to breathe. Learn how to use it for your benefit.

In a nutshell, this machine will help you breathe. You can't talk due to the tube in your airway. Your hands may be tied down, or, you may be heavily sedated so that you don't dislodge the tube. To get the spit out of your lungs you will have to be suctioned and this will take your air away too, but it will be replaced by the machine. Understanding this whole process can make it easier to cope and your ability to cope will play a large part in your getting off of this life support. Also, as a visitor, the better you understand the process, the more you can help someone you love to cope. **Please read a more in-depth discussion about the ventilator experience (pg. 132) in the Equipment Section.** Understanding this process could help save your life or the life of someone you love.

In addition to the ventilator you may need the life support of the same kinds of drugs used in emergency life support. Only now you may be receiving them as a continuous intravenous drip. At any time, one or more of these drugs may be the only thing keeping you alive. Please note that in some illnesses such as Sepsis, a potentially life threatening body reaction to an infection, many doctors will give you these life support drugs and *not* consider them to be *code drugs*. This is important to understand when you have made yourself a No Code, which we will talk about soon.

Some drugs or devices that you have been using in your routine daily life could become life support, things such as insulin, dialysis, internal pacemakers/ defibrillators, antibiotics, tube feeding, etc.

So, in critical care you can be using any or all of the above drugs and equipment to keep you alive until your body can heal. I like to think of it as "Life Support *Therapy*". This is therapy to get you over a bump in your road of life. To me it is "therapy" until it crosses the line. Whose line? **Your line**. Also, it is "therapy" until we reach a point where it is only postponing inevitable death. We'll talk more about this in chapter 3.

LONG TERM LIFE SUPPORT

If it is possible and available we will provide long term life support until it doesn't work anymore or you or your family say to stop. That is the way it has been in the USA. It may not be that way in the future.

If for some reason you're unable to breathe well enough off of the ventilator, you may stay on it for months, a year, or maybe even for the rest of your life.

If you need the ventilator for longer than about ten to 14 days, you will have a hole surgically cut into your windpipe so a tube called a *tracheostomy* tube can be inserted (See equipment chapter for more detail).

If your heart is not working properly, you may need an *internal pacemaker/defibrillator.* Or you may need a *ventricular assist device* (VAD) to keep your heart pumping. Or maybe it's all under control with drugs.

Maybe you need *dialysis, frequent blood transfusions, insulin, antibiotics*, etc. If you're unable to eat, for example, due to a coma, stroke, intestinal issues, cancer, etc. then *artificially providing you food and fluid through a tube* into your stomach, or an IV line into your veins is another form of life support.

You can see there are many everyday drugs, technologies or diets that we take for granted that can become life supports.

You can use these drugs, diets and technologies to extend your life for a while and then, if your quality of life declines to a place you don't want, you can stop using them. Once again, knowing *where **you** draw the line* will be important. It's important that you know your rights and that you are still in charge. Even if you become unconscious or mentally incompetent, if you have taken steps to understand and communicate your wishes effectively you will be in charge. We'll discuss this more in chapter 6.

CODE STATUS

Okay, now that you know where you want to draw the line, how much you'll pay, and how much you're willing to go through, you can decide what your CODE STATUS (resuscitation status) is.

Code Status describes how much or how little life support you want. **Everyone has a code status**. By law everyone in the USA is a FULL Code unless a person has written otherwise.

Being a **"Full Code"** means we will use all of our know-how, drugs, technology, and procedures to keep you alive no matter what.

In a **"Limited Code"** you specify which life supports you want to use. It's your *customized* mix and match code status. For example, you can say it's okay to put you on a breathing machine (*intubation and ventilation*), but don't shock (*defibrillate*) your heart or press on your chest (*compression*) to make your heart pump. Or maybe you say it's okay to do compression and shocking, but you want none of the machines for breathing.

You have to understand what you are asking for. Your body needs to take in oxygen and blow off carbon dioxide and it needs a working pump to circulate all of that. So, if you say "yes" to the ventilation but "no" to compression or shocking, then your body will be getting oxygen but it will not be circulating it because the heart is not pumping. Vice versa, if you say "yes" to compression and shocking, but "no" to the ventilator, your heart may be pumping but we may not be able to give you enough oxygen to keep your organs alive for very long. Another thing to consider are the drugs. Maybe you are okay with the drugs, but, you don't want compression, shocking, or ventilation. We may be able to give you only drugs successfully in some situations.

But, we may not. Again, if your heart is not pumping, they will not be getting circulated.

You can have what you want, just please, understand what you want.

You can be a **"No Code" (also called DNR – do not resuscitate)** and refuse all of the supports. No Code refers to the life supports of CPR, defibrillation, intubation, and life support drugs.

I want you to understand that when you make yourself a No Code you can specify FULL CARE or COMFORT CARE depending upon your condition.

No Code/Full Care refers to *no resuscitation.* It means you do not want compression, shocking, ventilation, or drugs to stop your body when it is trying to die. Until that time you still receive your normal medical, surgical, emotional, and physical care.

For example:

You could make yourself a No Code at age 18 and you will still receive all of your usual healthcare unless

1. You get into a situation where you need emergency resuscitation, or

2. You have become terminally ill and your body is trying to pass.

No Code/Comfort Care can be started when your body is near passing and we are talking about "end of life" care, or, we are withdrawing life support. In this situation, we stop trying to force your body to stay alive. At this point you may stop artificial feeding, antibiotics, oxygen, etc. We still take good care of you and will provide pain meds, anti-anxiety meds and other comfort meds. Our focus becomes your comfort and allowing your body to have a peaceful passing in its own way and time. (See Palliative/Comfort Care, below).

ALSO I want you to be aware that, as I mentioned earlier, even if you have made yourself a No Code, some doctors do not consider the life support drugs called *pressors* to be a "code-type" drug in a Sepsis situation. So you could end up on one or several of these drugs to keep you alive while your body fights an infection. That is perfectly okay IF that is what you wanted. In my experience, some people do not want us to try to stop their body from dying when it is trying to die and they see being in septic shock as a *"window of opportunity"* to let go and have a peaceful passing. If you are one of these folks, you need to make sure you communicate this and do your paper work effectively. More of this in chapters 6 and 8.

Now, you can start out as a Full Code and use life support as long as you can, or you can try the life support for a while to see if it can help you get over a rough situation, then if it seems you aren't going to recover to a level of functioning that is okay with you, you can change to a Limited or No Code.

On the other hand you can start out a Limited or No Code and change it to Full Code. Your code status is actually fluid and can depend upon how you or your family is perceiving or coping with the situation when it is happening. (See the stories in chapter 8.)

PALLIATIVE CARE/ COMFORT CARE

I want you to be aware of the difference between *palliative care* and *comfort care*. The reason this is important is because it is often the same doctor that offers both services. And *that* is important because a person who is in pain but not ready to let go and have a peaceful passing may be afraid to talk to a palliative care doctor. This is because they are afraid that doctor is actually treating them with the intention of a peaceful passing. Please know that, yes, there can be overlap, but, they also can be totally different services.

Palliative Care is medical or surgical treatment that is intended to relieve pain and promote comfort. In my ICU we often called the Palliative Care team to help find good pain control for a patient, who is *not* dying,.

On the other hand, Palliative care *is* commonly used in terminal illness, *not to cure* the illness, but to relieve discomfort; for example, surgery, radiation, or chemotherapy being used to *reduce* the size of a tumor but not cure it. So please do not suffer needlessly because of fear. Just be very clear with the doctor of your intentions.

And on that note, when your doctors, whether they are cancer doctors, kidney doctors, brain doctors, or heart doctors, are offering therapy, ask them if it is *curative or palliative*. This will give you a clue as to whether or not they think they can *actually cure* you or if it is *just to buy more time*. Knowing this might make a difference in your choices.

If you're a No Code and it is the end of your life, you won't have to endure pain, difficulty breathing, or fear. You can request Comfort Care. With Comfort Care you'll be given medicines such as pain meds, anxiety meds and other meds to help keep you comfortable and allow you to have a peaceful passing in your own time.

So, do you want to be a Full Code, Limited Code, a No Code/Full Care or No Code/ Comfort Care? Do you know? Do you know the code status of the people you might have to make decisions for? Remember, everybody has a Code Status. In an emergency situation, if we have no idea what you want, we are obligated by law to do it all.

Please keep reading.

6

COMMUNICATION
(effective Living Wills, POAs, EMS No CPR, and POLST)

So, you've decided on what kind of disability you can live with / your basic level of functioning/ where you draw the line, and you know your desired Code status. You know how much you're willing to go through, and how much you're willing to pay. Now you need to communicate your wishes. You need to tell your spouse, your significant other, your kids, your parents, your doctor, and anyone else who might be *involved* in making major health care decisions for you. Even if your family lives in other parts of the country, let them know your wishes. You'd be surprised how a serious illness will bring people out of the woodwork and to your bedside.

On the other hand, if *you* want to know what your loved one's wishes are, don't go up to them and say "Hey mom, what do you want to do about dying?" Instead, try this approach: "Hey mom, I've been thinking about what I would want done if I should ever become really sick or injured. I realized that if I was unconscious my family should know what I would want so they could follow through with my wishes. Then it occurred to me you might have thought about this for yourself. Have you? Do you have any wishes you want me to know about?"

Another example is a person who, tried to talk with her father about his wishes, but he would never answer her. So she said to him, "Dad, you won't answer me, so I am going to tell you what I will do if I ever have to make health care decisions for you. If you don't like what I say, you better speak up and tell me what you do want." He never did tell her and in the end, she made the decisions she had told him she would do. She felt good about her decisions because he had never told her anything different. However you approach the subject, try to promote a loving discussion.

Sometimes expressing your wishes can be a stumbling block. It's important that *you* know where *you* draw the line. If you are unsure or wishy-washy about your wishes, your family will feel that you really don't know what you want, and then, if and when the time comes to make decisions, they won't know what to do. Or, maybe, your loved ones and even your doctor might not agree with your decisions. You may need to assign someone *outside* of your family the power to make healthcare decisions for you if should you be incapacitated. If your doctor doesn't agree with you, you may need to find another doctor. Remember, your family and your doctors are people with their own beliefs and desires. You need to give them love and respect while getting your own needs met.

This is also a time when you, as family, need Unconditional Love to allow the person you love to have the life experience they want. I'm sure because you love this person, you will want to keep them with you for as long as you can, in almost any condition. You are probably willing to do whatever it takes to take care of your loved one. It can be very hard to remember it isn't what *you* want that counts, it's what your loved one wants that matters. If necessary, seek help to work through all of the issues. I am hoping this book will be of help to you and your loved ones.

Hopefully, you will have been able to have these discussions with your family. Whether you actually talk to your family or not, you need to make things as clear as possible, so the first thing you should do is fill out a *Living Will,* or an *Advanced Directive.* (These two forms are essentially the same thing).

LIVING WILL / ADVANCED DIRECTIVE

To help your healthcare team and your loved ones to understand your critical care and end of life wishes you should fill out your Living Will or Advanced Directives and discuss them with your loved ones and your doctor.

These forms can be as simple as one page or many pages long. Whatever you use, try to get one that has a place where you can write down a *customized statement* of exactly what you want. (one patient wrote it down in the margins.)

Most of these forms come with generic statements that you can simply check off "yes/no". The simplest statement will basically indicate, "Yes, do everything to keep me alive."

The other may say something to the effect of: "If at any time I should have an incurable or irreversible condition caused by injury, disease, or illness certified to be a terminal condition by two physicians, and if the application of life-sustaining procedures would serve only to artificially postpone the moment of my death and if my attending physician determines that my death is imminent or will result in a relatively short time without the application of life sustaining procedures, I direct that those procedures be withheld or withdrawn and that I be permitted to die naturally."

This is a fine statement but I cannot tell you how many times a family member has brought this to me at the patient's bedside and it is not helpful at all due to its vagueness and being subject to interpretation. This is one of the reasons I have written this book.

Carefully read and consider these prepared statements. The above statement draws the line at an incurable or irreversible condition that will cause death within a reasonable period of time. This is a very *vague* statement. I cannot tell you how many times the doctors have differing perceptions over what is terminal or incurable.

Does the statement tell us what level of disability/ basic level of functioning you are willing to live for? Does it express where *you* draw the line for quality of life? Is "terminal" where you drew **your** line? What if you may not be terminal but, according to medical experience, there is a high probability that saving you with life supports will eventually leave you with a disability that is below your acceptable basic level of functioning?

Does the statement tell us what kind life support you are willing to have or how long you are willing to have it to achieve your bottom line?

Don't hesitate to customize these prepared statements. Feel free to add to them or to cross them out completely and make your own statement. For example, on both her Advanced Directive and DPOA one woman had crossed out the prepared statements and had written down in the margins, "Don't give me life support for any reason. Don't give me CPR, no defibrillation, no intubation, no life sustaining drugs, no food or fluid, only give me the comfort care of pain medicine and tranquilizing medicine, and let me have a peaceful passing." This lady knew what she wanted. She didn't believe death was the end of life; rather, she called it, "My Life... Part Two: The Adventure Continues."

Done well, this document can give us a clue and provide good guidelines to direct your care if you're incapacitated.

DURABLE POWER OF ATTORNEY FOR HEALTHCARE (DPOA)/MEDICAL POWER OF ATTORNEY (MPOA)/HEALTHCARE POWER OF ATTORNEY

Too often a very ill or injured person comes to the critical care unit only to have family and friends disagreeing and arguing, about what the person really wants. This is why a good Advanced Directive is so important. Sometimes they get into a competition about who is going to make decisions. Due to everyone being focused on their own grief, competition, and the potential of losing you, they often choose what they want for themselves rather than what you wanted for yourself.

In addition to your Advanced Directive it would be wise to fill out some kind of *power of attorney for healthcare*. The form is about your **HEALTHCARE**, not your estate which deals with your money, property, etc. States use different names for essentially the same type of form. These are some of the names of the forms I am talking about: ***Durable Power of Attorney for Health Care (DPOA), Healthcare Power of Attorney (HPOA), and Medical Power of Attorney***.

All of these forms are "state specific" meaning if you currently have a DPOA done in one state and move to another, you need to fill it out again on their paperwork. You can get all of these forms for free at many places including your doctor's office, hospitals, the Area Agency on Aging, the Internet, and, for a price, in stores that sell business forms. A good place for state-specific forms and other helpful information is on line at **http://www.caringinfo.org**.

In these forms you are assigning someone to be your spokesperson (*surrogate*) in case you are so ill you are considered incapable of making healthcare decisions for yourself. You give this person the power to make health care decisions including life and death decisions for you. This spokesperson needs to sign the form indicating that he/she *agrees* to make decisions that *follow your stated wishes*. Making these decisions for someone you love is hard. Make sure the person you choose is capable of doing the job. I've seen too many DPOA's who cannot stand up to the pressure given them by other family members, doctors, or nurses. You need someone who can be your champion! To help your DPOA, tell the other folks, who may be concerned with your healthcare, what you have decided and that you have made this assignment of a DPOA.

If you are incompetent, you are totally alone in the world, have family disputes about you, or, if no other surrogate can be found then the state can be asked to appoint a guardian for you. In Washington State this is called a *Guardian ad litem;* in other states a *conservator.* This is a court appointed guardian to make healthcare decisions for you. This may be a professional guardian or someone in your family who meets the qualifications of guardianship. For example, I knew a woman who went to court to get guardianship of her grandfather who was incapacitated from Alzheimer's. She did this because her mother, the patient's daughter, was not taking good care of him. The court acting in the patient's best interest granted the granddaughter guardianship.

A guardian, legally, has more power to make decisions about your healthcare than anyone else. The legal power to make decisions is usually as follows in descending power:

1. The appointed **guardian/conservator** of the patient.

2. The person to whom the patient has assigned the **power of attorney for health care** to make healthcare decisions.

3. The patient's **spouse**. In some states neither "same sex" relationships nor "common – law" relationships are counted as a spouse. So, if you want

your partner to have rights to make decisions for you...*make them your DPOA!*
  4. **Adult Children** of the patient
  5. **Parents** of the patient.
  6. **Adult Siblings** of the patient.
  7. Some states add more to this list

It does not matter, *legally*, if a person who is lower on the list does not agree with a person who is higher on the list and has more legal authority.   Also, if the decisions are to be made by multiple children, or two parents, or multiple siblings then some states *require* that everyone within that specific "level" has to agree and give a unanimous decision e.g. – *all* of the siblings, or *both* of the parents. Other states will allow the most competent person in that level to make decisions. Others go by who is oldest.

Even though legally we are to follow your surrogate's decisions, if there is disagreement among the significant others, even if your desires are written down, the medical staff *may* not let you go. We want to avoid causing more trauma to your family. We will try to help your family and friends by educating them about your situation; by helping them work through their denial and grief so that all of them can come to agreement and, hopefully peace, about the decisions being made

The people making the decisions need to resolve their differences and come to an agreement.   The important thing for all of these people to focus on is what their loved one would want to experience.

Bottom line – make it easy on your loved ones, do the paperwork and spell it out!

Another issue is if, for some reason, your surrogate suddenly decides to NOT follow your wishes *we will know this because you have written down where you draw the line/ what kind of disability you are willing to live with/ what is your acceptable basic level of functioning!* In a case like this, we *can* disregard the errant surrogate and follow your written wishes.

Just as a precaution, if you know there will be someone who will go against your wishes, make a note on your advanced directive that says, "Don't listen to Aunt Mary; she doesn't have my best interests at heart." Just give us a clue!

Also, be aware that once you have been pronounced dead, your DPOA's authority over your body stops and, unless you say otherwise, your body is then part of your estate and decisions are made by your heirs, etc. So, if you want to do something special with your body, like cremation, organ donation, autopsy etc. you need to write this down in your Advanced Directive and give your DPOA the power to make these decisions too.

Another issue I've noticed during my lectures is that our elderly seniors seem to have the perspective that no one would bother to put them on life support at their age. I hate to tell you, but I have personally taken care of people in their late 90's and early 100 years of age who were on life support and the family wanted it that way. Maybe this is what the person wanted, maybe not. It doesn't matter how old you are, you must think about these things, decide, and communicate.

You can easily do this paperwork yourself, but, if you foresee problems in your family, then it might be a good idea to have a lawyer help you. You can still make it a customized statement.

EMERGENCY MEDICAL SERVICE - NO
CARDIOPULMONARY RESUSCITAION (EMS – NO CPR)

In Washington State, in the past, when a person definitely did not want resuscitation, they could ask their doctor to fill out a form called an EMS – NO CPR form. This form told the emergency medical services *your wishes* to not resuscitate you if had no pulse or you were not breathing. You were supposed to wear an EMS - NO CPR bracelet to identify you to the paramedics, EMTs etc. This was a good initial attempt to meet people's wishes. But the problem was that often when people had this form done they didn't understand that in order for the EMS to follow it the person had to have *stopped* breathing or to have no effective heart rhythm. It did not stop you from being put on a ventilator because you were *just having difficulty* breathing. It did not stop you from having your heart paced because it was too slow. It did not mean you would be a NO CODE, receive comfort care, and allowed to die have a peaceful passing. There have been a number of times when elderly or terminal folks who thought that when the time came they would pass peacefully actually ended up in critical care on a ventilator and still wearing their EMS - NO CPR bracelets. Fortunately, Washington has a new form called a POLST. If you have an EMS - NO CPR form, it will still be honored but remember its drawbacks. I recommend you replace it with the POLST.

PHYSICIAN ORDERS FOR LIFE SUSTAINING TREATMENT (POLST)

The Physician Orders For Life Sustaining Treatment (POLST) is appropriate for any person, including a Full Code, but, it is especially good for anyone who wants to be a NO CODE, or LIMITED CODE.

The POLST was created in Oregon where it has been widely used. It has since been adopted in several states and is currently being considered in more states. The EMS throughout the state of Washington have been trained to use it. It is a brightly colored form and easily recognizable by the EMS. In Washington State it is bright green. In California it is a bright pink form.

The POLST does not replace the Advanced Directives or your DPOA. You still need to know what you want, talk to your family, assign a spokesperson, fill out your forms and talk to your primary care provider about your wishes.

What makes the POLST so awesome is that they are **doctor's orders** that reflect your wishes. The doctor actually writes down orders that can be followed by the EMS and hospitals regarding how much care you want. The form spells out all of the "code" care in detail. It tells us whether you are a Full Code, Limited Code, No Code want comfort care, antibiotics, or artificially administered food and fluid. It tells who this form was discussed with, for example, you or your surrogate. Both the doctor and you, or your surrogate, needs to sign the form. The document can be filled out by other healthcare workers but then it has to be signed by your primary care provider (your doctor, nurse practioner, PA) to be effective.

ALSO, the POLST is always where you are. If you live at home, the POLST is with you on your refrigerator. (That's a good place; you can leave it bare or put it in a red envelope to help the EMS recognize it).

If you go to a nursing home, adult family care home, hospice, etc the POLST must go with you to be valid. Fortunately, the DSHS approves of the POLST as long as your care facility has a policy and procedure (P&P) on how to use it. (So ask your care facility if they have P&P's and are using the POLST.)

If you come to an emergency room or an acute care hospital, the POLST comes with you. Tell the nurses and doctors you have a POLST. Each place you go to can make a copy of your POLST; but, *you must keep* the original. Your POLST should be reviewed every now and then and must be reviewed if:

- you want to change it.
- if there is a significant change in your health status; or
- if you get transferred from one care setting or one care level to another.

Different care facilities will have their own "window of time" in which the POLST must be reviewed. If it isn't reviewed within that time period it will be invalidated. So make sure you the patient, or you the surrogate, ask to review your POLST form if you get admitted to a hospital or transferred to another facility.

As I said, the POLST is a new form so you may need to ask your healthcare providers if they know of it and are using it. I anticipate that this POLST or some variation of it will become the standard of care throughout the United States eventually.

When you have filled out your paperwork give copies of your written Advanced Directives, DPOA, and your POLST to your doctor and your surrogate. Always have them on hand to bring to the hospital each time you go. The reason is because even if you gave them to the hospital on your last visit, they will be in Medical Records and we may not have easy nor timely access to them and you may end up in a situation you did not want. To help avoid this be sure to always have your currently valid (if you have made changes) POLST form because, remember, these are actual doctor's orders which can and should be followed by the EMS and ER staff.

Sometimes emergency room personnel will ask, "If this person is a No Code and doesn't want life support why did he come to the Emergency Room? This is a ridiculous question. All Emergency rooms should have an area where people who are No Code can go for comfort care only. Then having relieved the suffering, the doctor, patient and family can decide whether this person should go home on continuous comfort medicines under the guidance of hospice, or whether this person should be hospitalized to receive this care. Every acute care hospital should have areas that provide for comfort care only. Our job is not only to promote healthy living but to also ensure healthy, peaceful passing.

Be sure to check with your local emergency medical service about where you need to keep the forms, especially the POLST, to ensure the EMS "first responders" will find them. By "first responders, I mean your firemen, ambulance service, police, etc, those folks who respond first to emergency calls. Sometimes they like the forms to be in a red envelope on the refrigerator or even in a plastic bag in the freezer.

THE BEST INTENTIONS...

Hopefully, the POLST will prevent resuscitation mistakes, but the reality is people often change their mind in an emergency. Or, you may be in the shopping mall when you collapse and a Good Samaritan will resuscitate you. The bottom line is whether or not you want life support, there is a big chance you or your loved one will end up in critical care on life support. That's the bad news. The good news is that you can still be in control whether you're conscious or not. How? Because you *have thought* about where you draw the line. You *have talked* this over with your loved ones and your doctor, and you *have written* down guidelines. What has been started can be stopped. However, now that you're here, you might want to re-evaluate your Code Status. If you had wanted to be a No Code, and now are on life support maybe you'd be willing to continue if it could get you over a rough spot and return you to your usual level of functioning. Or, maybe you were a Full Code, but now that you're experiencing life support you decide that you don't really want it. (see stories in chapter 8)

Now you need information.

7

WHAT'S THE SCOOP?
(how to ask the questions?)

You should frequently evaluate your progress. If you're unconscious, your family should be doing it for you. Try to get the big picture by asking the experiences of your doctor, the nurses, the respiratory therapists, the physical therapists, the social worker, etc. To get further information about your problem, your family can use the Internet, go to the library, even ask your friends. You'll get a broader picture of the possibilities, and it'll help you make decisions.

When you ask the doctor, nurses, etc, questions about your loved one's prognosis, phrase your questions this way:

- **"In your experience, how have you seen patients in the condition progress?** Have you seen them get off of life support?"

- **"In your experience, have you seen people in this condition get to a place where they can..."** Ask about *whatever your bottom line* was i.e. recognize their families, talk, eat, go to the bathroom by themselves, etc?

- **"In your experience how long have you seen it take to achieve this level of functioning?"** Did it take a month, several months, a year, more to get to your bottom line?

By asking for your caregiver's *experience*, you can get a clearer answer because they don't feel as if they are being put on the spot and having to predict what will happen *specifically* to your loved one. They're just telling you what their experiences have been with similar cases. This is a good thing because every case is both similar and unique. Remember to compare their answers with where your loved *one drew his line.*

Whenever you have a *gut feeling*, or just intuitively know something is not right, ask questions. Insist the staff explain things to you in a way that you can understand. Insist they convince you that things aren't wrong.

And remember that doctors and nurses are just people. Sometimes they're overworked, very busy, or feeling a lot of pressure and can't spend the quality time they'd like to spend with you.

Some are jerks. Sometimes you just can't communicate with your doctor or your nurse. Perhaps you just don't like or trust them. If that happens, you request a new one or get some mediation between the two of you. If you decide you don't want your doctor anymore, you must get a new primary doctor. One woman recently in the hospital had, a year prior to admission, decided that she didn't want her doctor anymore, but she hadn't told him or her insurance company. He was still listed as her primary care provider.

This doctor still had the right and the responsibility to come see her, to write orders for her care and get paid for it because she had to have a primary care giver. If you feel that you are not getting satisfactory care, change your care givers; if needed, speak to the Medical Director; or, if the problem is related to nursing, the Charge Nurse and so on. Go to the Hospital Administer if you need to.

Also remember, that your doctor is human and has his own beliefs and life experiences that will affect his perspectives. He will have his own ideas about what's right or wrong and might not agree with your decisions. If this is the case, you may need to hire another doctor. If you keep your doctor despite his disagreement, then you and your family may have to be prepared to battle it out with him. If there are disagreements, most hospitals have an **Ethics Committee** that you can ask to hear your case. This is a group of volunteers, doctors, nurses, social workers, chaplains, and others from many walks of life. They listen to the case from both yours and the doctor's point of view. They can make recommendations about what they think should be done, but currently, they don't write orders. This may help. If not, you can always go to court.

When you know you'll be seeing your doctor be prepared with your questions. I'm sure many of you have experienced having a ton of questions for the doctor and then forgetting them the minute he walks in. One patient had a great system. Every time she had a question, she wrote it down on a little yellow post-it note. She wrote one question per paper, and stuck it on the edge of her bedside table. When her doctor was making rounds, he'd peek into her room to see how many post-it notes were lined up and then adjust his routine to have plenty of time to talk with her. She also wrote down the answers as he gave them. It worked great for her. Also, if possible, have a third person with you, either a family member or your nurse. They might hear something you didn't. If needed, you can request that a **"family conference"** be scheduled with you, your family and as many of your doctors and primary care nurses as can be available. In this way you'll have their undivided attention. You have the right to have them spend time with you to give updates and to answer questions.

When you're trying to communicate to your doctor about a problem or symptom, try using the **Pain Scale method**. This system of *rating* a symptom and the effectiveness of treatment is a good way to describe any problem you are having, be it pain, diarrhea, stiffness, colds, whatever. Using pain as an example here is how to use it:

To describe your pain level use the numbers zero to ten, with ten being the worse pain you've ever experienced, then pick a number that describes your current pain level. As you take drugs or do things to decrease the pain, rate how effective it is by how the number changes. This way instead of watching the clock, you listen to your body. I usually encourage patients to regulate their pain medicine to keep the number below two if possible. When the number is higher, or starting to climb, take your pain med. If your medicine doesn't lower the number you have to ask yourself if:

1. **You've waited too long before taking it**. If you wait too long you may need twice the amount of

medicine to get it under control. Like a flower blossoming, pain will grow, unless you nip it in the bud.

2. **Was the dose too small?**

3. **Was it not given often enough?**

4. **Was it simply not the right drug for you?** I once had a patient who got no relief with Percodan but great relief with Percocet. They both had the same narcotic, but one had Tylenol and the other had Aspirin.

If you use your number system, you can figure this out and communicate it to your doctor. You say, "Hey, doctor, my belly is hurting six on a scale of zero to ten. I take my pills, and it still hurts six out of ten." Or, "The pain goes down to four, but then it comes right back up to six after a half hour. I need a better medicine." Or, "Doctor, my diarrhea was 8 out of 10, but after two Imodium it dropped to 2 out of 10." Doctors and nurses understand this kind of communication.

If you have good pain control you'll still hurt when you cough or move around, but the pain will decrease after you've settled down again. Whatever you do, make sure you keep your pain under control. We no longer want you to be toughing out the pain. Today we know about neurochemistry and the damage stress causes. If you're hurting, your brain will release stress chemicals instead of healing chemicals. Treat your body like you would treat a child that you love. It will help it get better faster.

In critical care, it would be useful for you to know what kinds of things, *indicators*, to look for in measuring his progress. Ask your nurses and doctors which specific indicators they are watching in your loved one's particular problem. Keep a little journal of these indicators. You'll be able to track the trends. In ICU patients often take steps upward then downward. Watch to see if the trends are "up / down, up/down" but steadily going **up? (getting better)**, or "up / down, up/down" going downward.

Depending upon the type of problem your loved one has, the following are some of the indicators you could keep track of. (See the equipment section for discussions of some of these issues.)

FOR PROBLEMS RELATING TO THE BRAIN:

1. Is there enough oxygen getting to the brain? No matter what your loved one's illness is, this is the ultimate question.

2. Is there a problem with increased pressure in the head? If so what's causing it and what's being done to relieve it? Keep track of the pressure readings.

3. Is there a problem or potential problem with bleeding? What is the cause: accident, aneurysm etc.? What is being done to stop, treat, and prevent further problems?

4. Are there seizures or vasospasms? What's being done to stop or prevent them?

5. What is the neuro status? How much of the higher brain is functioning? This is the part that makes us who we are. Is any dysfunction temporary or permanent? How may rehab help? *What level of functioning can be reached? How long will it take? Does it cross YOUR LINE?*

FOR PROBLEMS RELATING TO THE SPINE:

1. What level of the spine is being affected? Is there any decrease in normal functioning; i.e. decreased ability to breathe, decreased sensation, movement, bowel or bladder control, sexual function? Is it temporary or permanent? Will they need long term life support? *What level of functioning can be reached? Does it cross YOUR LINE?*

FOR PROBLEMS RELATING TO THE HEART:

1. Is it a heart attack or angina? Are the cardiac enzymes up? Do you need clot busting medicine? Do you need an angiogram; angioplasty, surgery, other therapy? Do you need some form of a stress test, echocardiogram etc? What is your Ejection Fraction – the amount of blood pumped out of the heart with every beat?

2. Is an adequate rhythm being maintained? Are intravenous drugs or technology needed to do this? What kind, how much, how long, are they working?

3. Can adequate blood pressure/circulation be maintained? Is fluid backing up into the lungs or the body? Are intravenous drugs needed? What kind, how much, how long? Is technology needed to maintain circulation? What kind? Is it temporary or permanent? Is surgery needed? Is a transplant needed? Is enough oxygen getting to the brain? *How will it affect the level of functioning in the future?*

FOR PROBLEMS RELATING TO BLOOD PRESSURE:

1. Is it too high? Are intravenous drugs needed or just pills?

2. Is it too low? If so, is it due to a problem with the heart? (See Heart)? Is it due to Sepsis, the body's reaction to an infection? (see Sepsis) Are antibiotics or antifungal medicines being effective? Are intravenous drugs (*pressors*) needed to keep a blood pressure high enough to get adequate oxygen to the brain and other organs? *How many* pressors are being used? Are they working? Are the pressors' doses so high they are *hurting* the kidneys or other body parts while trying to preserve the brain and keep the body alive? There is a limit to the effectiveness of these drugs; has it been reached? Is it time to stop? In the end, will there be enough damage done to organs to cause a *decrease in the level of functioning? Does it cross YOUR LINE?*

FOR PROBLEMS RELATING TO THE LUNGS
(You must read about ventilators in the equipment section):

1. How much oxygen is needed? How is it given: by nasal cannula, mask, or by intubation?

2. Is the machine doing all of the breathing, part of it or just supporting your loved one's own efforts to breathe?

3. What's your loved one's respiratory rate i.e. too fast, too slow, just right?

4. What's the volume of your loved one's own breaths, too low, just right?

5. How stiff (compliant) are the lungs? How much pressure does it take to get air into the lung?

6. How much sedation does your loved one need to get good ventilation? Is this due to ill lungs or to his inability to cope? Is all that sedation causing problems with lowering his blood pressure so much that it is hurting other parts of the body? (see blood pressure, above)

7. Can he cough out the spit in his lungs? Does he need suctioning? Is there a lot of spit/fluid?

8. What is his oxygen saturation (the amount of oxygen circulating in his body)? Is it high enough to help the organs? Is there enough oxygen getting to the brain?

9. How are his blood gasses, i.e., the acid-base balance? (see Acid Base Balance.) How is the Lactic Acid level?

FOR PROBLEMS RELATING TO THE KIDNEYS:

1. Is he making urine? Is it too much or too little?

2. If it's too much, is it a problem with the head, hormones, or blood sugar?

3. If it's too little, is there a blockage to the urine coming out? Is there something wrong with the kidney itself, or is there not enough fluid being circulated to the kidneys (Due to one of the heart/blood pressure problems)?

4. Does he need some kind of artificial filtering like dialysis, CVVAH, etc.? Is it temporary or permanent? Will he lose a kidney? Need a transplant?

5. How's the acid base balance? (see explanation in equipment section.) How are the BUN and Creatinine levels (lab tests that show kidney function)?

FOR PROBLEMS RELATING TO THE GI TRACT:

1. Any bleeding? If so, does he need blood or blood products? Procedures to diagnose and stop bleeding?

2. Any pain, yellow skin or eyes, swelling in the belly, feet? What is the cause? Is it affecting the blood pressure, circulation, kidneys, or brain?

3. Any nausea/vomiting? How is he getting nutrition?

4. Is he pooping? Too much, too little; is it normal color and, consistency, and odor?

5. Are all of the organs functioning within normal limits? If not, ask your doctor or nurse which tests are indicators that you should keep track of? It just depends upon the organ involved.

6. Does he need surgery?

OTHER ISSUES:

How are the electrolytes (salts) and sugar in the body doing--sodium, potassium, magnesium, calcium, glucose, etc.? Does he need replacements, does he need insulin? What is the blood count doing? The White Blood Cell Count indicates infections and the ability of the body to respond. How are the Hemoglobin and

Hematocrit? These help keep track of bleeding and anemia. How are the PTT or PT and platelets doing? These keep track of the ability to clot.

These are just some common tests. Remember, you need to ask your doctor and nurses *which tests are indicators for your loved one's specific illness.*

I just want to mention here that critical illness can raise you blood sugar, even if you are not eating, due to the body's stress and to medicines you are receiving. Having a normal blood sugar can help you to heal faster. So, even if you are not diabetic, you may find yourself having your blood sugar checked every hour and receiving Insulin injections or even a continuous IV of Insulin. It doesn't mean you will now be diabetic.

If you *are* diabetic you may find all of these same things happening to you, so, please don't be alarmed by the changes in your regime during this time period.

8

STOPPING LIFE SUPPORT

You must stay informed so you can track the progress of yours or your loved one's situation. Always compare the answers you're getting *with where you draw the line/what disability is okay to live with/ what basic level of functioning is desired.* Many times you'll come to a fork in the road where you will have a **"window of opportunity"** to choose to continue life support therapy or to stop it and create a peaceful passing.

One patient, a heart attack victim, upon whom CPR was not started soon enough, arrived at the critical care unit unconscious. There, his blood pressure and heart rhythm were controlled and, over the next week, he stabilized but didn't regain consciousness. Brainwave tests showed that he wasn't brain dead, but his brain functions were seriously impaired. The family was told that although this man may be able to come off of the life support and be able to breathe on his own in a few days, he had extensive brain damage. Right now he was in a coma, but he would probably come out of it and could possibly recover to a point where he would be alive, but he would need total physical care and likely he'd not recognize his family. This was a *window of opportunity*. Stop life support now, and he would pass away peacefully. Continue and he would be facing extremely limited recovery. There was conflict in the family; the wife and one son did not believe the Dad would want to live with such diminished capacity. The other son said, "We should give him a chance." In further discussions it was revealed that this son and his father had not had a great relationship, and only recently had begun working things out. This son wasn't ready to let go. In helping the son with his personal wishes we kept asking what would his dad want? If we give the dad this chance, would he have the capability and more importantly, the *desire* to face this challenge? He finally decided that Dad would not want to do this. This family chose to stop life support and allow a peaceful passing.

Most of us have heard of heroes who have faced the challenge of disabling injuries or illness. Some are famous, like Christopher Reeves and Stephen Hawking, but most are the people next door. When life gave these people poop, they turned it into fertilizer, and grew. You may even know someone who became a happier person within himself and in his life because of the changes the disability made. These people personify the strength of the human spirit. You can never discount the strength of a person's spirit and will to live. Every nurse has seen people recover despite the odds. These recoveries are called miracles because they don't happen every day.

Yet, when you are making decisions for someone else, it's very important that you remember it's *that* person who has to experience everything it takes to live, and you need to know whether or not this is a challenge that he or she would want. Too often we save people with life support and then they have to live with results they did not want. They are forced to face challenges they didn't want. Society has adopted the adage, "You don't know your own strength until you are tested", thereby making it *right* to face every challenge that comes our way. This implies that a person is weak or cowardly if he elects not to accept the challenge. This is simply not true. People should be able to choose those challenges they want to face and those they don't. It's the individual's choice rather than society's. Just because we can keep someone alive, does that mean we should?

Some answers I have heard regarding Technology are:

- God gave us technology to help us live.
- God gave us technology so we can play at being God and learn wisdom.
- God gave us technology so we could have a choice. Then when He calls us home we can go joyfully, or we can whine and say "Aw, do I have to come now? Can't I stay out and play a little longer?"

It's always hard to set aside your own feelings and make a decision based on what your loved one would want, but it's even harder if your loved one never told you what to do. Whatever decision you make, you must live with. You'll always wonder if you did the right thing. When you make a decision based upon Love and what you think your loved one would want, it does help you to cope in the future.

On the other hand, if your loved one *did* tell you what he wanted, how wonderful is that! This was a final gift of Love he gave to you. So, *know* that you aren't making the decision; you're simply honoring the decision he made; you're following his wishes. This is your final gift of love to him.

If you're conscious when you fall ill, you can always change your mind and override your written desires.

This is an excerpt from my other book, I May Be Crazy, But It's All Good:

"I want to tell you a different sort of story now; it doesn't have any spiritual communication in it, but, I so love it and I hope you do to.

It is about Lola.

Lola was in her 40's. She had a neuromuscular disorder that had been developing over time, making her weaker and weaker until eventually it would be fatal to her. Prior to being admitted to my hospital she'd already had a tracheostomy in place that she could plug and still be able to talk. She had known she would need the life support of a ventilator for breathing eventually; but, even at this stage of her process, she was not holding back on living her life to the fullest.

Fulfilling a lifelong dream, she and her boyfriend were en route to see the Grand Canyon when, in respiratory distress, she had to come to my hospital. Initially, she was put onto a hospital ventilator and then had progressed to being put onto a ventilator that she could use at home.

By the time I met Lola in the ICU, she had been on the home vent for a couple of weeks and wasn't progressing in large part because of her anxiety, depression, and agitation. She was requiring a lot of sedation to relax her enough so that the machine could assist her in breathing. She couldn't talk anymore. When I went to her bedside I saw her face was pinched into such a frown. Although, she was moderately sedated, she was still tense.

I said to her, "You don't look too happy."

She shook her head "No"

"Are you saying you are not happy?"

Nodded, "Yes."

"Are you in pain?"

Head shook, "No."

"Trouble breathing, too cold, too hot...?" I went down a list.

"No." She shook her head to all of the questions. Then she reached up and touched her trach.

"Are you unhappy with being on the ventilator?"

"Yes." She nodded.

"I was told you knew you would be on a ventilator some day and that this is what you wanted. Isn't that right?

She closed her eyes and shrugged her shoulders.

"Lola, are you happy with that decision now?"

"NO."

"Have you changed your mind?"

"Yes."

"It's okay to change your mind. You have a right to do that."

She moved her hands, searching for paper and pen. She wanted to write something. "Too late," she weakly scribbled, "I am on the machine."

"Do you feel stuck?"

She started crying and nodded, "Yes."

"Lola, you are not stuck, it is not too late. Yes, you are on life support and, yes, you still can choose what you want. You are conscious and alert. You are still in control of your healthcare. You can choose to continue on life support and have the best quality of life you can make; or, you can choose to stop life support, go on comfort care, let nature take its course and have a peaceful death."

Her eyes widened hyper-alert with hope. She grabbed my hand squeezing it tightly and nodded yes.

"I support you in whatever decision you make. I have a question though. Are you looking to escape? Are you sure you don't just need some more time to adapt to a new life style?"

"No, not escape." She wrote. "Grip reality. I am dying."

"But you knew that."

"Yes and been living life fully. Been happy. But crossed a line now. Now not being happy. Am holding on, resisting my death."

She stared at me to see my reaction. I nodded for her to continue. She seemed to become more alert, almost excited. Her writing became stronger, clearer.

"With my illness I learned to embrace life, let go of the usual expectations and I was happy. Now I want to embrace my death. Bring love and happiness to it. Am I a quitter, crazy, failure? I don't feel like one. It feels right but I don't want my daughters to be angry with me for going."

"Ahhh. I got it. You are an awesome woman. You have a lot of wisdom, thanks for sharing it with me. I am going to help you as much as I can. Okay?"

She smiled and nodded.

"Okay, the first thing you need to do is to be calm. You have needed a lot of medication to calm you down so the machine can help you breathe. Begin embracing where you are right now and stop needing these meds. You will need to communicate your wishes to your daughters and the doctor and no one is gonna believe you if you are depressed, anxious and drugged out. Understand?"

Nods.

"When you are completely drug free and calm, please re-evaluate what you are saying you want. You might not think the same way then. If you decide this is the path you want and you can demonstrate that you are awake, alert, calm, and coping, then talk with your daughters. They are going to need you to communicate your wishes from a place of love, not defeat, and somehow you are going to have to be able to do that. Can you do it?"

Smiles.

"Once you have convinced them, you will have to convince the doctor that you are completely aware of your choice and that it is truly what you want. It's gonna take a few days and effort on your part. How do you feel about it?"

She drew a smiley face.

Well, it took more than a few days. Lola's daughters got it right away. They knew their mom. They felt the love. No problem. Some of the nurses were having a problem, thinking it was an assisted suicide. I shared my perspective that there is a difference between withdrawing life support and assisted suicide. In the former, a body that has been *kept alive by artificial means* is finally allowed to have a peaceful death. In the latter, a body that is still *naturally alive but suffering* is helped to peacefully and comfortably die. This made sense to them and they became comfortable with Lola's decision. The doctor, however, was sympathetic but unsure. He insisted she have a psychiatric evaluation by not one doctor, but two. They finally all agreed that Lola was in her right mind, clearly understood her choice, and had a good attitude. They were impressed with her calm, certain presence.

Me, I was inspired by it!

Once she got the "go ahead", Lola began planning her death just like she would plan a birthday party. The friends and family she wanted to be present were notified. Her minister was notified. I brought in a beautiful aerial video of the Grand Canyon, but, first, she wanted a particular personal video to be played for everyone.

We moved her to the largest room in the ICU. People showed up and had their private times to speak with her. Then we watched her video of a benefit her friends had thrown to raise money for her trip to the Grand Canyon. It was a party with food, drinks, and a live band. The video centered on a particular dance. While the band played "Unchained Melody", person by person would drop money into a jar and take a turn dancing Lola around the floor. Male or female would tenderly put their arms around her and she would look at them with eyes and face glowing in love.

Oh my God, I don't think I can handle this!

It was all I could do to not fall apart. Tears were dribbling down my cheeks as I watched this video. My throat ached from choking back the emotion. I am the nurse, I am supposed to be strong, be professional!

I was a wimp. I was being overwhelmed with the emotion. Then I heard Lola's voice in my head, *"Don't resist... embrace in love and happiness."* I grounded and centered myself. I allowed myself to feel the pain and grief and to embrace it until, finally, it moved through to peace and then to love. Without resistance it just flowed naturally to love.

We never got to the Grand Canyon video. She had seen all she wanted - the love shared by herself and the people in the video and the love she was sharing right now with the people in her room. She wrote to me that it was time. I started the intravenous medications that would keep her from experiencing the anxiety that would come with shortness of breath. The intent was to keep her mind and body at peace when we stopped her life support. She drifted into a light sleep. I disconnected the vent. At first, she frowned and grabbed her daughter's hand. Then I whispered in her ear, "You are free now to embrace in Love." She smiled, became calm and in a few minutes, holding both her daughters' hands she peacefully passed away.

It isn't that I had never had a patient die before this. I just had never had a patient consciously choose to stop life support and have a peaceful death. I had never seen someone try to convince their loved ones that it was okay, the right thing to do, and then support the loved ones while they processed and grieved. I had never seen such loving strength, certainty and patience.

I had never been so emotionally melted in a patient's case. I learned I could "go there" with my patients and families. I could embrace my humanity within my professionalism and I could become stronger, more compassionate, more of a rock for my patients and families to hold onto during their most vulnerable times. Lola had given me a gift, a gift I embrace still today."

****

On the other hand there was a lady with extensive cancer who had never sought treatment because she was afraid of hospitals. Her family and friends knew she didn't want to go to the hospital let alone have life support. But when she became very ill at home, having trouble breathing, her husband didn't know what to do, so he called 911. Of course the paramedics were obligated to intubate her.

She became conscious while on the ventilator and was terrified to find herself exactly where she did not want to be. However she responded very well to my teaching her how to work with the ventilator, learning her options, and finding that she was still in control.

She became very calm and decided to stay on life support while tests were done to verify whether or not her cancer was treatable at this stage. She knew she could stop life support at any time and she knew she had the support of her family, doctors and nurses. The tests came back showing her cancer was at a terminal stage and at that time she too elected to withdraw life support and have a peaceful passing.

One more story I have to tell is of an older woman who had had cancer and had become very sick. This woman wanted to stay alive no matter what and was willing to be on life support. Her son and daughter knew this and when their mom became unconscious and all of the caregivers were advising to let go, they did not. Well, mom recovered. They had one more great year with her and then once again she became very ill. And once again, the kids insisted upon treatment knowing this is what she would have wanted. We kept going as long as possible. When this woman finally did die her children had no doubt they had done everything that could be done and that they had followed her wishes. Whatever the wishes are, when you know you have done what your loved one wants, it helps with the grieving.

As noted in Lola's story there is a difference between withdrawing life support and assisted suicide. In one, the *body that has been kept alive artificially* is finally allowed to have a peaceful passing. In the other, a *body that is alive and suffering* is helped to peacefully and comfortably die. I remember another line from Tuesdays With Morrie where Morrie says, "Don't give up too soon, but don't hang on too long." Life is precious, yet death will happen. How much better it would be if we could have it be just the way we want.

In critical care when a person is taken off of life support they may pass right away or it may take a few days even a couple of weeks. It just depends upon the person's situation. Generally if someone has a breathing problem and the help to breathe, including oxygen, is taken away, they will not last very long, in my experience, a few minutes to a day at the most. On the other hand if life support is being stopped because the person's injury or illness has disabled them beyond "their line", say after a cardiac arrest, stroke or other brain injury, it may take longer to pass. Artificially provided food and fluids are stopped and only comfort care is given. In this way, the body that cannot take care of itself anymore will naturally shut down and peacefully pass.

If it will be more than a day or so, your loved one may be transferred out of critical care to a medical room in the hospital where the family and friends have more freedom to stay. Your loved one may even be transferred to a Hospice center if the hospital is associated with one. This is a good thing.

When you or your loved one has a terminal illness you may want to look into end- of- life care provided by Hospice programs. In my personal and professional experience, Hospice is a lifesaver in the care they provide not only to the dying person but to the family and friends as well. If you have the opportunity to be in a Hospice program, you are lucky.

You can get hospice care if your doctor certifies that you are terminally ill and probably have less than six months to live. If you live longer than that you can still get hospice if your doctor continues to certify you are terminally ill. You can come off of hospice if you or your doctor decides to take you off.

Medicare pays for Hospice. You have a team of people to take care of you, including your own doctor, a nurse, social worker, clergy, therapists, and trained volunteers. Hospice care can be provided in a care facility; a hospice center, or even in your own home.   If you are home, your friends and family will supply the main care, supported by the Hospice team. Medical supplies, equipment, and drugs are provided.

Remember you can still receive Palliative Care if needed. Palliative Care refers to whatever medical or surgical care you need to keep you comfortable, for example, a terminal illness caused by a growing cancer that cannot be cured but can be reduced in size in order to decrease pain. Or, if your terminal but need your appendix taken out...it can be done.

What Hospice does NOT do is try to cure your terminal illness. It is normal to be a NO CODE in Hospice and, eventually, when your body decompensates you will be given comfort care and allowed to have a peaceful passing.   You can get more information on Hospice by contacting your local State Hospice Organization (which in Washington State is 888-459-0438 or 509-456-0438) or by contacting:

The Hospice Association of America
228 7th St. SE
Washington, DC 20003
1-202-546-4759
www.hospice-america.org

9

VISITING

If you think being a patient is hard, wait till you're a visitor.

First, you have to deal with the visiting rules. These will vary from hospital to hospital, unit to unit, and even nurse to nurse. They may be as strict as walking through a metal detector and having only two people visit for 10 minutes every hour between 10 a.m. and 2 p.m. Or they can be as flexible as, "Sure your dog can come in to visit."

Despite having a policy, visiting rules are a controversy among nurses, due to each nurse's perception as to what is safe and healing for the patient and the whole unit. Please be patient with us. Always ask your nurse how she wants to handle things; it may change from hour to hour. She might be bending the rules and taking a lot of flak for her decision to let you visit, so please be flexible.

Almost all critical care units have a waiting room that has a phone with a direct line into the unit. You are supposed to call for permission to come in. As with visiting rules, the rule to call before coming in can be strictly followed or not. Again, always check with your nurse.

If you want to stay but are being told that you can't, please, first evaluate what is best for your loved one. If you judge that it's best for you to stay, tell the nurse. Go to the supervisor, the director of nursing, or the administrator of the hospital, if you need to. But first always ask yourself *what is best for the patient.* And remember there are other patients in the unit to be considered too. Many units are not set up to have visitors stay at the bedside. The beds may not be in private rooms, rather, only curtains separate them. Be aware of the limitations of your unit and try to work with the nurses.

Visitors can be a healing factor or a hindrance to the patient's well-being. The patient's response to a particular visitor's presence will often decide who visits and for how long. If the patient stays calm and can rest in your presence, this is good. But it's not good if he's continually trying to get you to "rescue" him, and he becomes agitated because you can't. Sometimes you might have to leave for a while. Always make decisions based upon what is best for your loved one.

Don't sit and stare at your loved one. He'll probably feel it. Instead read a book, etc. If he wants your attention he will do something to get it. Like a child that you are trying to get to sleep, he'll wake up, see you there, be reassured, and probably go back to sleep if you don't engage him. But, if you are staring or responding to his every eye opening or movement, then like a child, he will stay awake.

Patients too often feel like they have to be good hosts and take care of visitors. This can wear them out. Please encourage rest and if he cannot do it in your presence...leave at frequent intervals.

Your nurse may or may not want you to touch or talk to your loved one. Sometimes the stimulation can be harmful. Find out what she thinks is okay.

Some nurses want you to leave when they have to do a task or procedure with the patient. Some will let you help with the patient's physical care, others won't. It can be difficult to deal with the varying preferences of the nurses, so be flexible, and remember that each one is doing what she thinks is best for your loved one.

When a person is in critical care, he'll often lose all track of time and awareness of what is going on. He'll develop blank spots in his memory, or he will think he remembers but does not. This is true when he's very ill, also when he's had drugs for various procedures, or to help him relax. Some of the drugs cause an *amnesiac* effect. The family can play a valuable role in helping their loved one to integrate the time and experiences he's lost because of amnesia or a decrease level of consciousness. It's generally accepted that a person is affected by his experiences even if he isn't conscious of the experience. This can leave him with odd feelings that he can't explain. So, to help him fill in the gaps, it may be a good idea for a family member to keep a journal their loved one can read when he's able.

So t you won't get your hopes up, if your loved one is in critical care due to a complication of substance abuse, do not anticipate this will teach him a lesson and cure him. Uh, uh, honey. More than likely, he won't remember a thing about being there and will be ready to use again as soon as possible. Also, without a patient's consent it's not legal to take pictures so you can show him the consequences of his abusive habits. Sorry.

PART TWO

CREATING A HEALING ENVIRONMENT

The traditional Western approach to health care is if you can't see it, poke it, cut it, or measure it, you can't deal with it cuz it doesn't exist. That's the Western perspective, but there are billions of people both western and non-western who perceive other ways to promote healing. In the past these ways have all been called Non-Traditional. Recently, many are called *Complimentary Therapies* because they are used *in addition* to traditional Western therapy. The wise son of a beautiful patient once told me that the difference between Western and Eastern medicine is that Western medicine tries to fix flat tires, while Eastern medicine tries to take the nails out of the road. I think it is holistic to embrace both in Unconditional Love and to use whatever is needed and best for your Highest Good.

Whether using the traditional drugs, machines, surgeries, or the complimentary herbs, massage, acupuncture, crystals, feathers, music, aroma, touch, energy, etc., the most important factors in creating a healing environment are an **attitude of Unconditional Love, and an intention to allow the Highest Good to be**. These must be the foundation for all treatments.

Of course, because you love this person who is ill, you'll want to create a healing environment, but the closer your relationship is to the patient the harder that may be to do. It can be nearly impossible. This is because **to create a healing environment around you, you must have one inside of you**. That's hard to do when you're stressed out. This is when a relative, friend, minister, or your nurse can be very helpful. It only takes one person to step up the energy and create a healing environment for everyone in the room.

When you come to the hospital to visit someone you love, it's easy to get caught up in the drama and trauma that can be a part of the critical care unit. It is easiest for the person who is closest to the patient, the one who has the most to lose. You may have conflicting emotions between what is best for your loved one and meeting your own needs. You'll want things to be back to normal. You'll want your loved one to get well, to be able to function, to talk to you, and to know who you are. You'll be afraid and lonely, and at times you'll feel helpless and sorry for yourself. You may be angry and resentful that you are in this situation. You'll be worried about finances: should you get a job? If you have a job, should you go to work or stay at the bedside? How will you pay the medical bills? How much will the insurance pay? Who is taking care of your kids, home? You'll want assurance that you have been making the right decisions for your loved one. You'll feel guilty when your loved one glares at you angrily because you won't untie his hands or take out the breathing tube. When you are ready to leave, you'll wait for a sign that it's okay to go. You may not get one. Or, worse, your loved one may be upset because you are leaving. How can you go? What if he dies while you are gone? The guilt is immense.

There's a difference between watching a drama on the TV and actually being there. Not only will you be experiencing your personal concerns, you'll also be experiencing the *mood* or *energy/vibe* around you and you may not even be able to tell the difference. You'll feel the energy of your loved one and of the people taking care of him. You'll pick up on the energy of the rest of the unit and the mood of other visitors in the waiting room. The waiting room is a world all its own. The fear, grief, anger, plus the support and strength visitors can give to each other are palpable. What will you bring to this stewpot of stress and emotions? Do you match the mood of the whirlwind that surrounds you, or can you maintain a sense of self- awareness and choose how you want to feel? Will you be a healing factor, or will you become part of the problem?

I am talking about *mood matching*. You've all experienced entering a room full of people and felt tension there. You are picking up the *vibe*. You may not know why the room is thick with tension but you may unconsciously match the energy vibrations in the room and become tense yourself. Your fight or flight mechanisms kick in. Later you learn that there had been an argument between two people, or bad news given to the occupants of the room. You may unconsciously relate that event to yourself. If it has meaning to you, you may continue to match and be tense. If it doesn't have significance to you, your energy will change, perhaps you become sympathetic or start cracking jokes to ease the tension. You may turn the mood around and get everyone laughing.

Then they will have matched you.

When you lose self-awareness and unconsciously match someone else's mood, you lose self-control. You start *reacting* instead of *acting*. *You lose your ability to perceive a situation, assess your options, and choose the one that is best.* How helpful can you be to yourself or to anyone else?

Physics teaches us that everything is made up of energy. Depending upon its frequency/vibratory rate, it will manifest as gas, liquid, or solid. Thoughts and emotions are energy at another vibration rate. Spirit is another vibration rate. You can utilize this knowledge to choose which energy level you want to communicate or transmit on. When you visit with your loved one try to think and feel Love inside of you. In this way you *step up* your personal energy vibrations, and they will be transmitted to him. Your very presence will affect the vibrations in the room.

You can do this by preparing yourself before you enter the hospital. While you are parked in your car close your eyes. Imagine Unconditional Love as a little ball of light. Then look for it inside of your body. If you need to, imagine you are watching yourself on a movie screen in your mind and see where that ball of light is located in your body. It is ALWAYS there. You just need to look through the darkness until you see it, like a candle in the night. If you cannot find the candle then imagine reaching over and turning on a light switch in your body. If you have too much trouble finding it, then imagine a blackboard where you draw a figure of yourself and then take a colored chalk and put the dot of light in your body. If you just cannot *see* anything, then listen for a sound/feel/taste/smell that represents Unconditional Love to you. When you finally see the light, or other sensation, you may feel a release of some emotional tension. That's great. Now, focus on this light or sensation. Let it become the only thing you sense. It will fill your mind, and you'll begin to feel it in your body. Let it fill you. Always keep yourself FULL.

Be like a fountain that keeps itself full and let's everyone else have its runoff. Remember that you can't give what you don't have. If you are empty you are going to *need* and won't be able to give. Try to maintain the awareness of Love inside yourself and *feel* it.

As you enter the hospital, be aware of the energy there and how it feels differently from the way Love feels. As you interact with people, be aware of how the different emotions compare to Love. Focus on Love. Bring this level of energy vibration to your loved one and communicate it with your emotions, thoughts, voice, and touch. Bring Love to your loved one with the intention of allowing him to have his Highest Good. You can step up the energy of every drug, machine, or person caring for your loved one by stepping up your vibration. Just like playing a low C on the piano then playing it an octave higher, your vibration is higher, and just like tuning one instrument to another, if you can maintain the tone, others will tune to you. You set the mood; others will match you. You transform them by perceiving them as instruments for the Highest Good. Then trust and allow it to be so.

But how can you do this when someone you love is in a critical condition? You'll have way too many strong emotions that will prevent you from focusing on Love. You'll be acutely aware of your dependency upon this person to fill a place in your life. It's important that you allow yourself to experience your emotions in a safe way. If you try to be strong by controlling your emotions, you just become controlling. But, if you can constructively experience your emotions, you become truly strong. If you need to be alone to experience these feelings, be sure you set aside time to do this, often. If you need to talk to someone, arrange it. If you have no one, ask the nurse, and she'll have the social worker help you.

During your emotional time allow yourself to feel what you feel. It's okay. Ask yourself what is the worst thing that could happen? Experience the fear and grief this brings. Then ask, what could be worse than that? Keep going until you can't think of anything worse. Then ask yourself how you will deal with this "most worse" situation. Find a solution. If you can't think of one right then, work on it; ask others until you find a satisfying solution. Once you have solved this "most worst" issue, you will know you can deal with the rest. When I use this technique, I allow myself to experience my full range of emotions. I do whatever I need to, in my imagination, to release my emotions until I can perceive a clear, effective solution and come to an attitude of Love.

If one of your emotions is loneliness try using this technique to maintain a connection with your loved one. Arrange a time and space where you'll be undisturbed and get comfortable. Close your eyes. Now use your imagination and pretend that you can see your loved one. Maybe you'll see an actual figure in your mind, or a symbol, color, sound, smell, or touch. Whether you see anything or not, tell your loved one *everything you ever wanted to say to him.* Then *LISTEN.* This is important. Too often, even in real life, we talk and never listen. If you don't hear anything, then *pretend.* Put words into his mouth and *hear him say all of the things you ever wanted him to say to you.* Then you reply to this. And, again, listen. If you don't hear anything again, make up another response from him. Keep up the conversation in this way. Have another one the next day, and the next. Eventually, you will the clear the energy between you and you'll find that you hear things that you know you didn't make up. Then you will have made the connection, you'll be tuned in.

I have found this technique to be very effective for my personal use and in spiritually counseling my patients and their families. I use this technique to help my patients work through issues they are facing with their illnesses, and to help them make the transitions from life in the body to life out of the body. The results are usually very subtle, but, on occasion, they have been fairly dramatic.

Here are another couple of excerpts from my book, I May Be Crazy But It's All Good:

"One day I was assigned to a young boy named Sam. I don't remember his history, but apparently he'd been in the ICU for a few days, transferred to Pediatrics and now returned, comatose, to the ICU. He'd had some kind of head trauma and now was having seizures. His doctor said he had a very poor prognosis and wasn't likely to live. That is all of the story I had.

I walked into his room. For some reason I just stood there at the foot of his bed and, in my mind, I said, *"Hello." In my imagination I saw a blazingly angry boy.*

He was yelling, "I'll teach them! I'm gonna die and then they'll be sorry."

WHAAAT? Holy moly, what is going on here? Am I really seeing this? I have no idea, but I don't see how I could be making this up. Sooo, in my mind I asked him, "What's up with you? Why are you so angry?"

"I'm angry that my dad took me away; he shouldn't have done that. And I'm angry cuz my mother treats me like a baby."

Whoa; is this real? I don't know what the heck he's talking about. What do I do now? What do I say? Okay, Linda, calm down and just talk."

I told him, "Yeah you could teach them really good. You could hurt them bad; but, you're gonna hurt yourself even worse if you die. How old are you... 8, 9? If you just wait a few years, you'll be old enough that no one can tell you what to do. You can do whatever you want. You'll have your whole life to live. Wouldn't you like to do that instead?"

He actually listened. After a few moments he said, "Well I hadn't thought of it like that. You could be right, I'll think about it."

"Well, okay then." I let it go and started doing my nursing care of this comatose boy. I wasn't sure what had just happened and I wasn't sure what to do with it.

Later on, when his mom came to visit him, I started feeling this revved up energy inside of me. I don't know if it was fear or anticipation. I felt like I was going to erupt. I had a strong urge to tell her what I had seen, so, I said to her, "You know what? I was pretending in my mind that I was talking to Sam and, man, he was pissed off. When I asked him why, he told me he was angry at his dad for taking him away and angry at you for treating him like a baby." I held my breath and watched her.

She stared at me and then started crying. She sat down with her head in her hands and sobbed.

UH OH, now what? I put my arm around her and waited.

She told me that, shortly after Sam was born, she and his father had separated. Then his father had kidnapped him. After all this time she had gotten Sam back less than a year ago. She was so afraid of losing him again that she kept a very tight rein on him.

"I don't let him play with his friends after school. I know it bothers him; we are always arguing about it. He tells me I treat him like he's a baby. I know he is more mature than the average kid and needs more freedom, but I am so afraid of losing him again."

She turned to Sam, leaned her head against his and said, "I'm sorry."

That night, after I left work, Sam woke up. The next day he was transferred back to Pediatrics. I was off work for a couple of days, but, when I got back I went to see him. I walked into his room. He was sitting on the side of his bed with his back to me. His mom and her boyfriend were facing me. She smiled and said, "Hi."

I went to face Sam, stuck out my hand and said, "Hi Sam, my name is Linda. I was one of your nurses in the ICU."

He said, "I know who you are and I know what you did." Then he threw his arms around me and hugged tightly.

What??!! Oh my God, I am gonna cry! I don't know what to say or to think. What is happening here? All I could do was to hold onto him. When we parted, I looked at his mom and her mouth was opened. I gave

Sam another big squeeze, told him to take care and have a great life; then I left. Actually, I left kind of in a hurry. This was too weird.

What had just happened? Did his mom tell him? Did he remember...how could he? What does this mean? I don't know but it was a profound experience for me.

Hmm I think something is happening here!

Crazily, a couple of months later I was talking about this story to some friends of mine. It turned out they actually knew the family and told me Sam was happier, doing well, and, getting along great with his mom. She had released some of her fear and was letting him live life again. I thought that was cool, but, I tucked it away on the "I can't explain it" shelf in my mind."

****

Another story from my book is about Mrs. Dodds:

"Mrs. Violet Dodds was a woman who had ARDS and Heart Failure. She had been very ill for weeks and had little chance of surviving. But she and her family had never discussed what she would want to do about life support. They only knew she wanted her family around her when she died. So the family insisted she stay on life support. They would be happy if she could just survive even if she would be bedridden and in need of full care. They just wanted her with them. They did, however, make her a No Code so that if she got worse we could let her go peacefully.

She was married to Todd. Her adult children were Tony, Mike, and Madeline. They were a close and loving family. For some reason I always remember Violet as Mrs. Dodds. She was a very sweet woman, very graceful even in her illness.

After I say, "Hello" to a patient's spirit, one of the things I may do is to have them stand in front of a full length mirror in my mind. I have them look at the "truth" of who they are rather than what they have been believing they are. I am always amazed at what they see there. It's different for every person. I don't always understand what I see but it is an awesome healing experience for the patient.

Mrs. Dodds had been in the ICU for almost a month. She had slowly worsened until she was unconscious. *One Saturday morning, I was talking with her in my head about her body, herself, what she believed about leaving her body, etc. Then, I asked her to look into the mirror.*

Violet's reflection was of herself at around age 16. She had long hair almost to her waist. She was dressed in a kind of white shift or maybe a muslin type nightgown and she was barefoot. She looked so very innocent and sweet to me.

"Violet, you are lovely." She shyly smiled. Suddenly, I could see that she was in a little field filled with daisies. She sat down in the grass and started to make a daisy chain. "Violet, what do you believe happens when you leave your body?"

"Oh, I will go to Heaven, Linda."

"How do you feel about going there?"

"I will be going soon, I know that. I am not worried or scared, if that is what you want to know. I know I will be with my Father there. Truly, I am looking forward to leaving. My body is becoming just a shell now."

"That's beautiful. I am curious though, if you are ready to go, why haven't you gone?"

She sighed, "I don't want my family to feel like I have abandoned them. And..." she hesitated, and then whispered, "Linda, I don't want to be alone when I die."

Later that day, her eldest son, Tony, was visiting. Tony, from my perspective was the most conservative person in the family. He wasn't into "spiritual" stuff at all, so I didn't mention my conversation with his mom, except for one thing. We were standing at the foot of her bed and I asked, "Tony, would you feel abandoned if your mom died?"

His face got all soft and he said. "No. I know mom would never abandon us. If it is her time to go then that is how it is."

I clarified, "So it would be okay for her to go when it is her time. Do the others feel this way too?"

He said, "Yes, we all love mom and want what is best for her. We know she loves us."

Hmmm.

The next day, Sunday, Mrs. Dodds took a sudden turn for the worst. Her heart rate dropped to 30, her blood pressure dropped. She was clearly in a dying process. None of the family was there.

She doesn't want to die alone, Linda. I know, I know. Hurry up, call everyone.

I called, Todd. No answer. I called Tony. No answer. I called Mike. No answer. I called Madeline. No answer. No one was home! I left messages on their machines. Desperate, I called Madeline's office. Her boss happened to be there on a Sunday and said he would try to contact her.

Damn, I can't find anyone; I don't know what to do. She doesn't want to be alone! Okay, Linda, you're starting to panic, just chill out; ground and center. Breathe. Okay, okay, she is dying and there is no one here but me.

Although, I had another patient, I didn't want to leave Violet alone. I asked the other nurses to please keep an eye on my other patient. Then I went into Violet's room, stood at the head of her bed and said, "I'm here, Violet, you are not alone." I started combing her hair, massaging her head and sending her love. It was quite peaceful.

All of a sudden in my mind's eye, I saw this male like figure with huge wings float down through the ceiling reaching for Violet. Then I saw Violet, in the image of the young girl in her white shift and bare feet, float out of her body reaching and wrapping her arms around the angel's neck. He draped her body in his arms and they floated up through the ceiling. Dreamy eyed, Violet, never took her gaze from his face.

Wooo, okey dokey now! Never saw that before. I took a deep breath and kept combing her hair. Her heart was still beating, but she was gone.

Less than five minutes later, her husband arrived. I asked if he had received my messages, but he merely replied, "No, I didn't get a message, I just came." Then, in just the space of another few minutes, one by one all of her kids were there. No one had gotten a message, they were just showing up. As they came into the room and saw the monitor, they all knew what was happening and surrounded her bed.

I asked, "If you could say something to Violet right now, what would you say?" Each one had a little message for her. When they finished, her body died.

Each person then had a little private time with her. When Madeline finished her time, I took a chance and told her what I saw. Her face lit up with joy.

A few weeks later some flowers and a card came for me from Madeline. She related how, at the funeral, people kept commenting that she seemed so peaceful about her mom's death and she would tell them, "That's because I know my mom flew off with an angel."

A few years later, I was in a jury duty holding pen and I heard someone yell my name. It was Madeline. She told me she has never forgotten and how much it has helped her in her life."

Tuning in to someone spiritually and talking to them can be very effective. Remember, though, you're there to help them, not to nag them.

Although it is socially unacceptable in many situations, amusement is another very effective tool. Amusement can break the bonds of fear, grief, and anger and allow the light of Love to flow. I will tease, scold, hold, touch, tickle, praise, laugh, curse, and cry with my patients and their families. I use whatever will work to create a healing environment for all of us.

These techniques can help you to prepare yourself to visit. They'll help you contribute to a healing environment because you'll bring energy vibe of calmness and Love with you. You'll be able to act, not react, to the situations around you. I'm not saying it's easy to maintain this calmness. Sometimes things will happen that can be overwhelming. When that happens it's helpful to step back, or leave the room, and use your techniques to get yourself together again. Experience your emotions; ask, again, what is the worst thing that could happen; decide how you will deal with it. When you are ready, go back to the situation. When you've learned to cope with your own needs and desires, you can let go of judgment and fear, and you'll be able to have Unconditional Love. You'll be able to ask, "What is best?" or "What is the Highest Good?" for your loved one. This is the basis of healing. Healing does not necessarily mean a person will get well and be just the way you think they should be. Sometimes healing is to leave the physical body. You cannot be the judge of what is best for another person; you can only allow it to be.

If your loved one passes, it would be helpful for you to understand grieving, so that when you think you are going crazy you will understand this is normal. There are bereavement groups provided by hospitals, churches and social service groups that can be very helpful. If you are not a group type of person, you may want to see a bereavement counselor. If you are the type of person who doesn't like to seek outside help then I recommend reading at least one book about grieving so that you are familiar with the stages of grief, and, as I said above, you will know you are not abnormal for the way you are feeling, thinking and behaving.

PART THREE

EQUIPMENT AND RELATED ILLNESS

If you've been brought to critical care, you may wake up and not have a clue as to where you are or what's going on. Or, maybe you did know ahead of time that you'd be in critical care after surgery; you may have even been told that you'd be on a ventilator, with a lot of tubes and monitors, but the standard pre-operative teaching often really doesn't prepare you for what you'll *experience*, particularly the experience of being on a ventilator. Due to the drugs, you probably won't remember much of the worse stuff anyway, but even though you don't remember the experience, it's imprinted upon your psyche. This sometimes creates free-floating anxiety; something bothers you but your conscious mind doesn't remember what. That's why it's so important to keep you informed. I can count on one hand the number of people I have met who get *more* anxious when they get information. Most people want to know what is happening to them even if it is scary. If you don't understand what's going on, you may become frightened and fight whatever is being done. We are your partners in your health care. We need you to help us take care of you. It would be helpful if you better understood the critical care experience.

The following is a description of some of the equipment you'll find in critical care and some of the illnesses that require their use. **This is not a complete list for sure.** You'll find I go into more detail about those things that I often discuss with patients and families. Some of it needs to be read in sequence, some doesn't.

I want to mention first that you won't get much sleep in a critical care unit. Uncomfortable things frequently bug you, things like a blood pressure cuff squeezing your arm, catheters or IV's that irritate you, being poked for blood samples, x-rays being done, lights that are always on, constant noise from machines and people, nurse's cold hands, or being uncomfortable and unable to move. Procedures, baths, and medicines will disrupt your sleep. You need to ignore these things as much as possible and try to cat-nap. It's like being on the front lines in a war zone, your body is exhausted but your awareness is always on alert. It's almost impossible to get into the much needed "dream sleep" time. Some people will start experiencing ICU delirium. They'll begin to hallucinate due to lack of sleep. This is a serious problem and a patient affected by this problem needs to be moved out of critical care as soon as possible. It may take a week or more for their body and mind to trust that it's okay to sleep. Gradually the amount of time and the depth of their sleep will increase and their mental status will improve.

Another thing I want to mention is that you'll frequently receive medicines via your IV. Depending upon the kind of medicine and how fast it's given, you might feel yourself begin to "spin" or" float" out of your body. If you do feel this, *enjoy it, fly away and have a good time.* It's just the medicine and not something to be afraid of. People pay big money to have these sensations sometimes. You might also hallucinate because of your illness or because of the medicines. *Enjoy it.* The important thing to remember if you are hallucinating or floating is to not be afraid, instead have fun with it. If you are seeing ghosts turn them into Casper - type friendly ghosts. If you are seeing spiders, turn them into Charlotte's Web - type friendly spiders, etc. If you are visiting someone who is hallucinating try to turn it into something amusing for them. Fear creates a bad experience.

INTRAVENOUS LINES

You will have at least one intravenous (IV) site, but, usually a minimum of two in ICU. I know you don't want to be poked, but you are going to appreciate that we can give you fluids and some medicines and sometimes take blood out of this tube. It is all to help you. Some nurses have a gift for starting IVs. I call them *IV whisperers*. So, if your nurse is having a hard time, ask if one of these "whisperers" are around to help.

An IV is a small *catheter* that has a smaller needle inside it. The needle is poked into your vein then the catheter is slid over the needle and into your vein. When the catheter is in place the needle is removed. So, *remember there is no needle left in your arm.* Knowing this can actually reduce the perception of pain from an IV. This IV catheter may be capped off and held in reserve, or it may be hooked up to fluid. If you don't have fluid running in the IV, you will receive a small flush of a solution to help keep the tip of the catheter from getting blocked by a blood clot. Sometimes this solution stings; sometimes it doesn't.

IV's that are put into the smaller veins of the hands, arms, or feet are called *peripheral IVs*. Peripheral veins cannot receive all the fluids or drugs that we might need to give to you, nor can they receive fluids as fast as we might need to give them, and some drugs are very irritating to the smaller peripheral veins. Also, because it's good healthcare practice to help prevent infections, your peripheral IV sites will be changed every few days. You can quickly run out of peripheral sites. For all of these reasons, you might need to have a *central IV catheter.*

Central IV's are bigger and longer than a regular peripheral IV. They're inserted either into your upper arm, your neck, your chest, or your groin, and then advanced so that at least the tip of the catheter is in a large "central vein" of the body where there is more blood flowing. Here, drugs are less irritating, and we can push in fluid faster. These catheters may have one to three outlets that allow us to give you different fluids and drugs at the same time. They can also be used for taking blood, thereby saving you from being poked.

A common central catheter is the *Triple Lumen Catheter*. This type of IV still needs to be changed frequently, about every seven days.

Another common central IV is the *PICC*, or peripherally inserted central catheter. It will be inserted into a peripheral vein somewhere in your upper arm and then threaded into a large central vein. This type of IV, and others like it, can be kept in the body for a much longer time. This is great for long-term therapy, home therapy, and even in hospital use when someone needs IV access for more than a week, or just because they are a hard stick (difficult veins to get a needle into). Other long term IV access can be put in under the skin in the chest with minor surgery, but this is not usually an issue faced in the critical care unit. These are used a lot for chemotherapy.

The placement of all IV's is a sterile procedure, so you need to hold still. This can be challenging, especially with the lines placed in your neck, because your face will be covered with a sterile towel. Some patients get claustrophobic or have problems breathing under it. Just tell us if you're having a problem, and we'll try to help. Sometimes it can take a while to put these lines into just the right place, and we'll need your help and patience to work together to be successful. It will be worth it in the end because we can offer you so much more with these IV's.

BLOOD PRESSURE CUFFS/ARTERIAL LINES

You'll most likely have an *automatic blood pressure cuff* on your arm or your leg. When it squeezes it is looking for a pulse, so, if you are moving your limb it thinks it is a pulse and will squeeze tighter. It can really get tight and hurt. So when you feel it squeezing you should not move that arm (or leg), not even the fingers (or the toes), until the cuff has totally relaxed again. If you are visiting someone and notice that they cannot stop moving the limb or their fingers twitch, perhaps you can just gently hold the fingers or arm in place until the pressure is done. Check with the nurse to see if it is okay. These cuffs can be adjusted to squeeze from once a minute to every two hours or more. It just depends upon how closely we are monitoring your pressure. Most often they will go off every hour.

Sometimes instead of the cuff you will have a special IV-like catheter called an *arterial line* that is put into the artery of your wrist, your groin or your armpit. This line will be hooked up to an IV pressure bag and to the heart monitor where the pressure will be translated into an electrical waveform and numbers that tell us your real time blood pressure. Arteries are different from veins because they are under a lot more pressure. You must be careful to not dislodge an arterial line, because the artery can pump blood out of your body very fast, causing a big problem. You will love that we can take blood samples from this catheter, so you won't need to be poked. This catheter also allows us to monitor, in real time, the effects of certain drugs on your blood pressure, allowing us to fine-tune your meds.

HEART

Your heart is a bio-electrical-mechanical pump that has four rooms in it. The two top rooms are called the right and left *atrium* and the two bottom rooms are called the right and left *ventricles*. The blood comes from the body and goes into the top right room of the heart, and then it goes through a set of doors called *valves* and into the bottom right room. Next, it goes through more doors and into the arteries of the lungs where it gets rid of the old air (*carbon dioxide*) and picks up the new air (*oxygen*). After this, the blood goes into the top left room of the heart, through some doors and down into the bottom left room. Then it goes through more doors and out into the body via a big artery called the Aorta. The heart beats a standard range of 60 to 100 times a minute and pumps a standard range of 4 to 8 quarts of blood each minute.

In the top right area of the top right room is a group of cells (*the sinus node*) that act like a traffic cop. It's the main traffic cop and I call it the "Top cop". There is also "backup cop" (*the av node*) at the junction of the two top rooms and the two bottom rooms. The Top cop sends an electrical signal down routine pathways, first to the two top rooms, then through the backup cop to the two bottom rooms telling the cells in your heart to squeeze (*contract*) thereby pumping blood out. This is called a beat. So, first there is an electrical signal then a mechanical squeeze. The routine pathways are important because they keep the blood flowing in an effective forward flow.

Heart Monitor

You will be connected to a heart monitor. You'll probably be able to see your heart rhythm (*ECG*) on the monitor in your room. Ask your nurse what your normal heart rhythm looks like. Don't be alarmed if you sometimes see a bunch of erratic squiggles. You can make that happen just by jiggling the wires on your chest, moving, coughing, etc. However, it may be that you *do* have extra and/or different beats at times. If you notice you feel differently when you are having those beats, that's the time to call your nurse. But if it's anything serious, more than likely she'll already be there, because she can see your rhythm on the central monitor at the nurse's station.

As you get well, you may be connected to a portable heart monitor called a telemetry monitor. This will give you the freedom to be out of your room and still allow us to monitor your heart, but this only works within a certain range, so be sure to ask your nurse where you can go for a walk.

Pacemaker-External/Internal
Bradycardia/Blocks/Asystole

Sometimes the Top traffic cop stops telling your heart to beat and neither the backup cop nor any other cells take over the job and your heart just stops beating (*Asystole*). This is a Code Blue situation that needs life support and critical detective work to figure out a cause and how to treat if possible.

Sometimes, the Top Cop makes your heart beat so slowly (*Bradycardia*) that you cannot maintain a good blood pressure and consciousness. This too is a code situation and you will need some type of life support intervention. With Bradycardia you may be connected to a machine called an external pacemaker. You'll have extra heart monitoring wires attached to your chest that allow the machine to watch your top cop's signal to your heart. If it's needed, this machine will give little paced shocks to make the heart squeeze blood to the body. These shocks are uncomfortable, and you'll be given pain medicine and tranquilizers if necessary. You may need an internal pacemaker.

Sometimes the Top cop is sending out the right signal and the top rooms give a beat, but the signal gets *blocked*, partially or totally, by the backup cop. In this case the bottom rooms aren't getting enough signals to beat. In this case too, you may need a pacemaker. Stimulating your heart in this way might be temporary, or it may be the first step toward a *permanent internal pacemaker.* If you get a permanent pacemaker, it'll be a minor surgical procedure to insert it under your skin and connect the wires directly to your heart. You'll be restricted in moving your left arm for an amount of time determined by your cardiologist.

Cardioversion, Atrial Flutter/, Atrial Fibrillation/ Ventricular Tachycardia

As previously discussed, there is a traffic cop in the top right room of the heart that tells the heart when to beat. When this Top cop sends the electrical signal and it follows the routine pathways, the heart pumps most efficiently. However, actually every cell in the heart has an ability to start the signal that could start a beat. Sometimes, one or more of the cells in the *top* rooms will start a riot, causing the two top rooms to have very fast inefficient squeezing even to the point of just quivering. This could be either *atrial flutter* or *atrial fibrillation.* Fortunately, the backup cop will allow only so many of those beats to get to the bottom rooms. That's why this heart rhythm isn't always a problem, and people can often just live with it. The problem comes about when the backup cop gets so overwhelmed that it lets too many beats through. Then the bottom rooms start beating too fast. Remember that the heart is a pump, and it needs a time to rest and fill so it has something to pump out. The bottom rooms of the heart are the main pumps. If they are beating too fast they cannot fill enough, and this can cause your blood pressure to fall. That's when your top rooms get into trouble, your doctor may have you try a couple of good coughs to slow down the heart, or, drugs may be used to get the beats to slow down, or a machine may be used that can give moderate shocks (Cardioversion) to stun your heart and allow the main traffic cop at the top to take over again.

Sometimes one or more cells in one of the *bottom* rooms have taken over the beating. This is called a *ventricular rhythm*. If it's only one beat it's called a PVC (*premature ventricular contraction*) and it isn't really a problem. Lots of people have them their whole lives. If you have several PVC's in a row it's called *ventricular tachycardia* (V-Tach). This can come and go and may or may not require treatment. If it stays but isn't beating too fast nor causing symptoms like chest pain, shortness of breath, low blood pressure, etc., it's called *asymptomatic ventricular tachycardia*. Your doctor may try to control or change it with drugs only, or he may give your heart a shock (Cardioversion) so your main traffic cop can again take over. People often come to the hospital to electively have this procedure done. After the procedure they can return home.

Defibrillator- Internal-External/ Ventricular Tachycardia/ Ventricular Fibrillation

If that cell in your bottom room makes the heart beat too fast, you won't have a good blood pressure, and you may have chest pain, sudden sweating, and difficulty breathing. And you may pass out. This is when ventricular tachycardia is called *symptomatic*. This is a life-threatening situation. It could also be that not just one cell but a bunch of the cells in your lower rooms are having a riot and making your heart beat extremely inefficiently, just as described for atrial fibrillation. This is called *ventricular fibrillation*. It's similar to when the top rooms did it, but now there is no backup cop to control the rate. When the bottom rooms are beating erratically or just quivering, there is not an efficient squeeze to get blood out of the heart and into the body.

Either of these rhythms is an emergency life support (code blue) situation just like those you've seen on TV. You'll die if you do not receive resuscitation help. You need *CPR*, and you'll need to be shocked by a machine called a *Defibrillator* to stun those cells, so that, hopefully, your Top cop can get control again. You will need drugs and you will have been intubated during the code and then, once you are stabilized, you will be connected to a ventilator to assist with breathing. If your heart has this problem repeatedly you may need a little defibrillator put inside your chest. It's a minor surgical procedure just like installing the pacemaker. In fact, you could have a combination pacemaker/defibrillator. You may feel the shock when the defibrillator fires. Usually the shock happens so quickly it's done before you're aware it's happening, but there was one patient I had who could feel the charge building inside his chest, and he would start a soft cry that would crescendo into a loud yell as the charge built and shocked him. He'd had his device for several years, but his heart had continued to decline to where he was eventually being shocked many times a day. His distress was palpable to the nurses caring for him. Eventually, it became too much for him to live with, so he requested to have it turned off, knowing that he would die without it. And he did have a peaceful passing.

Heart Attack

Although your heart's job is to pump blood into the body, the first area it pumps to is itself. *(Oh isn't this just a great example of how you need to keep yourself full so that you can give others your runoff? - See PART 2).*

The heart muscle has three major arteries called *coronary arteries*. Each artery is like a big three lane freeway that brings supplies to the towns along its particular route. If you have partial blockage in one or more of the *lanes* on a freeway, you'll still get supplies through but not as much. If the whole freeway gets blocked, and there is not a good system of "alternative side roads" (*collateral circulation*) to get the supplies through then the towns along that route will die. The threat of death is even bigger if more than one *freeway* is blocked. Like the towns, your heart's cells will die without the proper blood supply. This is the *true* heart attack or *myocardial infarction*. "Myo" = muscle, "Cardio" = heart, and "infarction" = death. When this happens you will have pain that is called *angina*. This pain is typically felt over the heart and down the left arm, but you may instead feel it in your neck, jaw, back, right arm, or in the top part of your stomach, like heartburn. You might not have pain but just pressure, or nausea, or you may feel short of breath. However, not all angina pain means you have actually had muscle cell death; sometimes it just indicates spasm or irritation. So when you come to the hospital with a heart attack always ask your doctor, "Did I have muscle death or just irritation?" Irritated heart cells will heal. Also ask, "If I had muscle cell death, how much? How well does my heart pump now? What percentage of blood is pumped out of my heart with every beat (*ejection fraction*)?" This may improve some after the cells that didn't die, recover. This will help you understand the condition of your heart and why the doctors may be recommending a particular treatment.

If you have a blockage, there are certain clot busting drugs that you can receive, but, they are most effective if you get them within two hours from the moment you have symptoms. You should be sent right to the Cath Lab for some kind of artery opening procedure such as an angioplasty. Do *not* drive yourself to the hospital because, one, you could pass out and get into an accident; two, if you can get 911 help the paramedics may be able to start treating you right where you are at. This will save time and your heart muscle. If you lose too much heart muscle it will affect the pumping ability of your heart. This can lead to heart failure which will definitely change your quality of life.

Echocardiogram/Stress Tests

This is a simple test to see the pumping ability and blood flow in your heart. The machine bounces sound waves off of your heart and creates a moving picture for the doctor to see. While you lie in bed, the tech will put some Vaseline type jelly on your chest then slide a little scanner across your chest. You'll be able to see and hear your heart on the machine's screen. Another way to do this is for the doctor to put a tube into your mouth and down your food pipe (*esophagus*) to pick up the sound waves from inside your body thereby getting a closer look at your heart beating. Ask your doctor what your *ejection fraction* (EF) is. This the amount of blood your heart can pump out with each beat. Low EFs will definitely affect the quality of your life.

I just want to talk a little bit about stress tests. These are done to see how well your heart can function with activity. If you are able to do it, you will be walking and running on a treadmill. But if you are not physically capable of using a treadmill, you will be given drugs that stimulate the heart as if you were being increasingly active.

Sometimes patients get very uncomfortable and emotionally stressed when they are lying on a table, not doing anything and yet their heart is beating fast. I like to suggest that you close your eyes and imagine you are doing an activity you love doing; one where you expect your heart and lungs to have to work harder as you do it. Here is an example:

Mr. Jones had one leg amputated and needed to have a stress test. He'd had them before and hated the experience. I asked, "Have you ever enjoyed doing some kind of activity that would normally increase your heart rate and breathing?"

"Yes, but it's been so long." He glanced down at his stump. "I used to be a runner."

"Awesome. How about if you close your eyes and picture a place you used to love to go running and just start out at an easy comfortable jog. As you feel your heart and lungs going faster, imagine you are running faster and faster and enjoy the experience."

He looked at me a little weird, but nodded okay.

He test results were better than they had ever been and when we were done, he was elated.

"It was just like I was out there running again!!" a tear fell down his cheek. "I haven't been able to do that for so long. It was wonderful."

I know it is a cliché, but using the power of your imagination to create a "Loving and happy place" in your mind can help decrease resistance and allow whatever is happening to be a positive experience, contributing to your well beingness.

Angiogram/ Angioplasty/Stent

One way to see the condition of your heart's arteries is to do an *angiogram*, which is an x-ray type procedure where the doctor puts dye into the arteries of your heart and takes pictures as the dye flows through. This way your doctor can see where you may have blockages.

Your groin on both sides will be shaved for this procedure. The pulses in both of your feet will be marked with a felt tip pen. You'll be taken by gurney to the Cath lab in the x-ray department and slid onto an exam table. The lab is often chilly, so let the tech know if you're cold. Also, you'll be lying flat on a hard table. Tell them if you're uncomfortable because you're going to have to hold still once the procedure begins. You'll see some TV type monitors, and there'll be a C- arm type x-ray machine that can be moved over the top of your body. Sometimes this is just inches from your face. Sometimes you can see the monitors and watch the inside of your heart. You won't be put to sleep, but you'll be given medicine that will make you relax, and you may fall asleep. The techs are going to scrub your groin, usually the right side, and then put a sterile sheet over your body. From then on you must keep your hands down at your sides because everything on top will be sterile.   When the doctor comes in he'll use a medicine (similar to what dentists use) to numb your groin, so you'll feel a little sting.   After that you shouldn't have any pain. If you do, tell them. Next the doctor will put a short tube, like a big IV catheter (*sheath*), into your femoral artery which is in your groin and then insert a long skinny catheter through that until it gets into the arteries of your heart. Then dye is injected and, as it circulates, you might feel a hot flash. Some people have said it was very hot, others say it's just warm. Pictures are then taken of the inside of your arteries. They'll show if you have any blockages and any collateral circulation.

If your hospital and doctor are allowed to do *angioplasty*, your doctor may choose to do this procedure at this time. He'll take out the heart catheter and then, through the same sheath, he'll put in a different, long, skinny catheter with a balloon on it that can be blown up at the blockage site, smashing the fat against the wall of the artery thereby opening the artery. It would be like pushing a landside off of the freeway. The balloon does block blood flow and, briefly, can cause pain.

Sometimes, the doctor may decide to put a little metal device in the artery called a *stent*. It's a little wire mesh tube that will fit against the wall of the artery, make it stronger, and help keep it open, kind of like a concrete tunnel would do in a hillside. You may also receive an IV medicine that will thin your blood for the next several hours or so and then pills for an extended time.

When the procedure is done, the catheter will be removed and the sheath will be taken out either right then or when you've returned to the critical care unit. In the critical care unit, the nurse will put a lot of pressure on your groin to stop the bleeding. She may do this with her hands or with some type of pressure device. This can be painful. She may numb your groin and give you some pain medicine before she starts. Your activity will continue to be restricted. You won't be allowed to sit up or move your leg. The purpose is to avoid sending pressure to your groin and possibly dislodge the clot that is forming there. If you do, you'll bleed quite fast. So you must keep your leg straight, and don't lift your head. If you need to cough, sneeze, or vomit, please reach down and support your groin. The nurse will be checking your groin for bleeding and your foot for a pulse to make sure whatever clot is forming is not cutting off your circulation. Your cardiologist and the protocol of the critical care unit will determine how long you have to lie around.

Usually, it's at least six hours, but it could be all night. If you have back pain, be sure to tell your nurse before it gets out of control. If you need to pee or poop, you'll use a bedpan, or a urinal, or you'll have a catheter inserted.

Some doctors will take out the sheath while you're in the cath lab and either inserts a type of material that acts like a plug-in-the-dike or they'll insert a certain type of suture that stops the bleeding. These have varying degrees of success. But when they work it's great because you can be up in just an hour or so.

So, in a nutshell, your discomforts will be the cold, the hard table, the sting of the numbing medicine, the hot flash, when the balloon is up, the pressure to stop bleeding when the sheath is removed, and lying flat on your back in bed for several hours. Don't hesitate to ask for drugs or other therapies to help you get through this.

I know all of this can be a big drag, but truly, it will be worth it, because if you "pop your clot" you will have to start the countdown all over again. When you are told you can start moving again, feel your groin area and get familiar with it so that you can tell if there is a change. If the clot pops and you start bleeding out of the puncture site, you will feel fluid on your skin. You need to put pressure on your groin and call for help. If, you feel a bump/goose egg starting to form, this is bleeding *under* the skin (*hematoma*) and, once again, you need to hold pressure and call for help. If these things happen after you get home, you need to call 911.

Newer technologies are being developed every day to make seeing blood flow easier, for example, using CT or MRA scans. Check with your cardiologist.

Coronary Artery Bypass Graft (CABG)

Why would you need bypass grafting? As described in the Heart Attack section, if the supplies don't get to the towns (cells) in your heart they will die. If you have total blockage of your freeway and the towns it supplied have already died, there is no reason to create a new route, but, if you have only a partial blockage of your freeway you may get in a small amount of supplies to the towns that are still there hanging on by a thread. To help them get more supplies you need either a good system of alternate side roads for collateral flow, or you need to put in a new major route.

That's what a bypass does. The cardiac surgeon will take an artery or a vein from another part of your body and sew it into your heart, bypassing the block, so the blood can travel down a new route to feed the heart cells. This surgery can be a "big deal", but technique and technology is just zooming along and this surgery has become less threatening. In fact, I am always amazed at seeing a patient leave for surgery in the morning, come back a few hours later looking so pale, still asleep, on the ventilator and with tubes all over; then by dinner, they may be sitting in a chair eating!

Whether you have many little heart attacks or one big one, if you lose too much heart muscle your pump will fail. This is called Heart Failure.

Heart Failure

The heart is just a great pump. It pumps blood out to the body which then returns it back to your heart all via a network of arteries, capillaries, and veins.

Heart failure is a problem with the heart muscle and its ability to pump blood forward to your body. There are a variety of things that can mess up your heart muscle, including heart attack, infections, high blood pressure, radiation, chemotherapy, and some drugs, etc.

Depending upon the cause, the muscle wall may be:

1. *Too stiff* and *inflexible* to let the bottom room open and fill with blood. It is like the difference between trying to fill a tennis ball versus a balloon; the ball is inflexible and can hold only a small amount while the balloon can stretch and hold more.

2. *Too thick* so that there isn't enough space in the room to put blood. This would be like adding padding to the inside of a wallet; the walls are thicker, so there is less room for money.

3. Too *stretched* and loose, so it fills but has no strength to squeeze and pump out blood. This would be similar to the elastic in a pair of pants that has been over stretched and now cannot spring back into shape.

Still, the body continues to return blood back to the heart and this can create problems.

If the RIGHT bottom room of your heart is having the pumping problem, then blood will back up into your body. You will have swelling in your legs and too much fluid in your liver, your intestines, etc., causing bloating, decreased appetite, and pain in the right upper part of your belly.

If the LEFT bottom room of your heart cannot pump forward, then blood backs into your lungs and you have problems with breathing, especially at night when you are lying down. This is called *congestive heart failure*. If it gets really bad it will be called *pulmonary edema*, a condition where your lungs are flooded, and you are coughing out pink frothy spit. Either of these situations can be life threatening, and you may need to be intubated and put on a ventilator until we can help your heart.

To maximize your heart's pumping ability the doctor will try to control those factors that affect the pumping action. First is the *volume* of fluid the heart has to pump. It has to be just the right amount, not too much, not too little. Too little fluid is usually not an issue unless you've become dehydrated. The usual problem is too much fluid. Your doctor will tell you to limit your salt intake, and he'll give you drugs to make you pee. You'll also receive drugs to slow your heartbeat so your heart has time to fully fill. Remember the heart muscle has a certain amount of elasticity, like a rubber band. If you stretch a rubber band just the right amount it will rebound strongly. If you don't stretch it enough the rebound is weak, if you over stretch it, it loses its ability to rebound. By controlling how much fluid is in the heart and giving the heart time to fill, the doctor can maximize how much your muscle stretches. This makes the rebound stronger and helps the heart muscle to pump blood out.

Secondly, to maximize the strength of your heart muscle's ability to pump, your doctor will give you drugs that increase the muscle's strength and ability to *contract.* This increases your muscle's ability to squeeze out the blood.

A third factor is how much pressure the heart has to push against to get the blood into the body. This is called *resistance.* Imagine the difference between sending water out a 3-inch garden hose and a 1-inch garden hose. It takes a lot more effort to push blood through a narrow artery than it does to push it through a wide artery. So you will also receive drugs to help control the size of your arteries.

All of these therapies will decrease your blood pressure. People in heart failure have very low blood pressures, and they get use to this. If you need this balancing of fluid and drugs, you may need an IV catheter, called a Swan Ganz (PA) catheter until your doctor has found just the right balance for your heart. This catheter will be discussed later in this section.

Ventricular Assist Devices/ Balloon Pumps/ Heart Transplants

The failing heart will become progressively worse over time. Modern technology has created, and continues to create, machines to help the heart do its job. One such machine is called a *Balloon Pump.* It is a temporary device that decreases the pressure the heart has to pump against. This may allow a weak heart muscle to pump enough blood to keep your body alive until you can receive further treatment. At the same time it increases the amount of blood flow to the heart's own arteries to feed the heart muscle. When you're on a balloon pump you may or may not be in a very critical time. You may be on a ventilator and have a lot of life support drugs. You may or may not be conscious. You won't be allowed out of bed, and your movement in bed will be restricted so you won't accidentally dislodge the tubes. When you're stable enough, you may be able to go to surgery for bypass grafting.

When surgery is no longer an option, you may have a device inserted that will, in effect, substitute for one or both of the bottom rooms of the heart. There are several kinds of devices. One kind is called a *ventricular assist device* (VAD). This is a tube inserted into your bottom room, and the blood drains into a machine that is a *mechanical pump.* Eventually you may have a small mechanical pump inserted into your belly. The pump is wired to batteries outside of your body. This mechanical pump can be a temporary replacement until you have a heart transplant, or it can be a permanent replacement. You can go home with these devices and be up and around, but you need a 24-hour companion who has been trained in using and troubleshooting your heart pump. I have full faith that, unless a better way comes along, these pumps will get easier to use in the future. Technology just gets better and better.

If you need a *heart transplant* you need to know if you're a candidate for a transplant. Not everyone is. You must discuss it with your doctor. If you are a candidate, you'll need funding to pay for the transplant.

Check whether your insurance will pay for it. Some people receive donations from private parties or groups. There are whole teams of people and support groups available to assist you with information and help you through the process. Transplantation of any organ will take you through the whole menu of what critical care has to offer, plus it has its own issues of drug therapy and life style changes that I won't go into in this book. I *will* mention that I believe the use of a complimentary therapy based in energy work, such as Healing Touch, or Reiki, can help integrate the energy of the host with the new energy of the transplanted organ.

Swan Ganz/PA Catheters

These catheters are not used as much as they use to be, but, sometimes it's important to know what needs balancing: the pumping strength of the heart, raising / lowering your blood pressure (resistance), or increasing / decreasing the amount of fluid circulating in your body (See Heart Failure). Sometimes it is a delicate balance.

In these cases you will need an intravenous catheter that can gather data and provide this information. A common name for this is the Swan Ganz catheter. It is a PA (*pulmonary artery*) catheter. This catheter is usually inserted into your groin or neck region, and then threaded up into the large vein that goes to the top right room of the heart. It goes through that room and down into the bottom right room of the heart. Then it goes through that room and into the big artery of the lung where it sits. There is a small thermometer on the tip and a little balloon that can be inflated when we want to check pressures.

With this catheter the pressure in all of the rooms of your heart and your lungs can be checked. Plus we can do tests that tell us how much blood your heart pumps out every minute and with every heartbeat. If we take all of these numbers, and your blood pressure numbers, we can calculate whether you need more or less drugs and /or more or less fluid. This is very useful in many problems, such as Heart Failure. It may be necessary after some major surgeries. Sometimes we put them in just to check how your heart is functioning, and then take them out.

Only one actual catheter is inserted into your body, but on the outside it will divide into several sections called lines. Each line has a different function. Some are connected to IV's, some to pressure bags and some to monitors. You'll see little waveforms on the monitor that shows you the pressures. There can be a lot of lines, and you may feel like the meatball on a plate of spaghetti. You have to be careful to not pull the catheter out. It's okay to move, just ask your nurse to help. The lines always seem to get tangled, and we appreciate your help in preventing it. When we're checking your pressures, it's called doing your *hemodynamics*. Usually you'll be lying flat in bed, relaxing and not talking. Checking your hemodynamics will help us fine-tune your therapies to maximize your heart's pumping abilities and your circulation status.

ACID BASE BALANCE

Your heart's job is to circulate blood in order to bring supplies to the cells and to take away waste products. It dumps these waste products into the various organs of the body where they are processed, recycled or dumped. A lot of the waste products are acidic. The body has three systems of neutralizing these acids. They are the kidneys, the lungs, and a chemical buffering system that provides base (Sodium Bicarbonate is a base chemical). The cells need oxygen to do their jobs but if they don't get enough oxygen, they can use a backup system to do the job for a little while; however, it creates more acid. If the body can't compensate or get rid of the acids, the cells will eventually die.

Think of how a swimming pool needs to have just the right amount of chlorine in it, not so much that it hurts the swimmer, and not so little that algae can grow. The body needs to have just the right amount of acid for the cells to float in and to work properly. The healthy range is very narrow. If acid level strays beyond this range and isn't corrected, it can be life threatening. There are many reasons Acid/Base can become imbalanced: Pneumonia, bad asthma attack, prolonged vomiting or diarrhea, liver or kidney problems, diabetes out of whack, infections, bleeding, shock, etc.

The lungs, kidneys, and buffer system maintain a fine balance. If you start having trouble with your breathing, the kidneys and the buffer system will try to adjust the balance. If you have trouble with the kidneys, the buffer system and the lungs will try to adjust the balance, and so on. If one system is chronically out of whack the other two will try to pick up the slack. This is why we can still live with so many chronic illnesses. But, when the systems cannot do their job, you will get sick very fast and will need us to use our know- how and technology to stand in as a substitute player to help your body get back into balance if we can.

LUNGS

Coughing and Deep Breathing

Your lung's job is to exchange old air (*carbon dioxide*) for new air (*oxygen*). The Lungs are like two apartment buildings with airway vents, rooms, and hallways. The airway vents are your windpipe (*trachea*), large air tubes (*bronchus*) and small air tubes (*bronchioles*). The rooms are the little air sacs (*alveoli),* and the hallways are the *blood vessels*. The lungs bring oxygen into the body and down into the little air sacs where the blood vessels pick up the oxygen and leave behind the carbon dioxide it brought from the body. The lungs then breathe out the carbon dioxide and the blood vessels bring oxygen to the cells of the body.

When you're up and around and breathing normally, you are fully expanding your lungs, so your airway vents are open, the doors of your rooms are open and the hallways are exchanging old air with fresh air. But when you're lying around, sick or in pain, your lungs don't fully expand, so your rooms collapse, the doors close and your hallways can't exchange old musty air for fresh air. This is called *atelectasis* and can lead to *pneumonia*. If you're not exchanging enough oxygen and carbon dioxide your body won't work right. The Acid – Base Balance will be off.

One of the best things you can do to help yourself is to routinely cough and deep breathe. Take six to ten huge breaths, as big as you can to open your rooms to air. Then do a couple of big, big coughs to blow open the doors of the rooms. And I don't mean one of those wimpy throat coughs; I mean a "he-man big belly" cough. Whether or not you have anything to cough up, the important thing is to keep those rooms and doors open.

But don't overdo it. Don't wear yourself out and cause your breathing muscles to get tired or hurt. Instead, watch the clock and pick the same time every hour to do your coughing and breathing exercises; for example, every hour on the hour. If you fall asleep and miss your exercises, do them when you wake up, and then start again on the hour. If it hurts you to cough, after surgery for example, be sure you hold where it hurts and give it support. Also, be sure to use your pain medicine properly so that you can handle the pain and yet not be so sleepy you cannot participate in getting yourself well.

Your oxygen levels will be intermittently or continuously monitored using an oxygen saturation monitor.

Oxygen Saturation Monitor

A little device will be clipped to your finger (or toe, ear, etc.) that will monitor how much oxygen is going through your body. The device sends out a red light that goes through your finger and gets picked up on the other side. The change in the red light allows the computer to calculate how much oxygen is circulating in your blood. You'll see this on the monitor as a waveform (pulse) and a number. This waveform and number are easily made inaccurate by several things, like how the device is situated on your finger, your blood pressure and circulation, how cold you are, and whether or not you're moving around. Before you can begin to trust the numbers, certain requirements have to be met that show the machine is picking up properly. Just ask your nurse to show you what reliable and unreliable waveforms look like. Then if you are watching it and it seems weird, ask your nurse about it.

One interesting thing to me is that when it is all working right, the sat probe's waveform represents the pulse. So when you look at the heart monitor you will see one line from the ECG that is showing the *electrical stimulus* for the heart muscle to squeeze and then the line from the sat probe shows that the *squeeze* happened. One time, I was working in an ICU and could see the ECG tracing working fine on the monitor, but, the sat probe was not showing it's waveforms. There can be a lot of reasons, as I have said, for this to happen. But, this time, when I checked, the patient actually *did not* have a pulse and was in an emergency (Code Blue) situation.

Nasal Cannula

If you need oxygen you'll receive it primarily from a nasal cannula. This is a tube that will go around your ears, under your chin and then into your nose. Some people complain that this tubing has an unpleasant odor, though most don't seem to notice it. Oxygen can be drying to the nose, especially high amounts, so tell us if you are experiencing any discomfort. We may be able to add a little water to humidify it. Also, they can eventually be sore on your ears, so let us know if this is happening to you.

This way of receiving oxygen is often enough for many people in critical care.

Oxygen Masks

If you need more oxygen, you'll need an oxygen mask. All the masks fit over your nose and mouth. Some have holes, some don't. Some have dials, some have plastic bags attached. Each type can deliver certain amounts of oxygen. At the top level is the *non-rebreather mask*. This mask has a reservoir bag on it that's filled with pure Oxygen. It has one-way valves that allow you to inhale the oxygen, but it won't allow your exhaled air into the bag. Also on the mask are one-way valves that let your exhaled breath out into the room but won't allow the air in your room from entering the mask. In this way you can get close to 100% oxygen. If you need this mask, you're having breathing problems and need more help than a regular mask can give you.

If you are wearing a mask and trying to put something into your mouth, i.e. food, fluid, pills, *don't take off the mask!* You need the oxygen! Just lift an edge and slip the straw, spoon, etc in under the mask. Just remember, BREATHING COMES FIRST! When your body needs to breathe, it doesn't care that you are planning on swallowing something. If you swallow and your body wants to breathe, it will inhale that stuff right into your lungs (*aspiration*). So hold the item in your mouth and swallow in between breaths. Do NOT eat or drink so much or so fast that you get your swallowing and breathing out of synch. If you cannot do all of this safely then you should not be putting anything into your mouth. The risk is too high for choking, aspiration, and pneumonia. Please be careful.

CPAP/BIPAP

You may need oxygen to be pushed into your lungs under pressure, or, you may need pressure to help keep those little rooms in your lungs open, or, both. You may be able to get away with using a special mask connected to a machine that pushes air into you. These are called BIPAP or CPAP machines.

These masks are put over either your nose, or your nose and mouth, and fitted very tightly to your face with straps that go around your head and under your chin. This is done so that all of the air goes into your lungs and won't leak around the mask. If you have a "nose only" mask and you try to talk the air going in your nose will come out of your mouth. Initially, these masks and the air being pushed in under pressure can be uncomfortable and have a steep learning curve, but once you get the hang of it, it can provide a lot of relief.

I tell people a story I read once about how dogs like to stick their heads out of the moving car's window. They love the wind blowing on their faces. I read it is because they pick up scents this way. So, try to imagine you are doing something you love to do that includes having the wind blowing on your face, for example, sailing or riding a bike. Then when the machine is blowing that air into your face, just suck it in and have a good time.

People with sleep apnea benefit greatly from these masks. Sleep apnea is a condition that causes people to intermittently block their breathing while they are sleeping. These people do not usually get restful sleep and over the years, they get used to never feeling rested. They also tend to snore, so their sleeping partners may not get much sleep either. It can be scary to sleep next to someone with sleep apnea. You tend to hold your own breath while waiting to see if your partner will breathe again.

The BIPAP/CPAP machines make it easier to breathe. Sleep apnea patients feel safer when they sleep, and both they and their bed partners can actually get a good night's rest. These machines are used at home and, frequently, in critical care they may be used to avoid using a ventilator if possible.

Ventilator

Ventilators are the life support for breathing. You may only need it for a few hours due to surgery, but if you're having trouble with ventilation, that is, you can't take in enough oxygen, release enough carbon dioxide, or safely cough out your spit, you will need to be intubated and put on a ventilator.

Many people need this help just to get over a rough time in their surgery or illness. You may need it for only a day, or it could be a week, or more. You may be conscious or unconscious.   However, it is still life support, and during that time, you may not be able to live without it.

The better you understand how to work with these machines the easier it will be for you to cope. Coping may decrease the amount of anxiety and sedative medicines you need. This could lead to less time spent on a ventilator and decrease the chance of secondary infections.   Coping will also decrease stress on your blood pressure and your heart.

Ventilators are machines that can either assist you to breathe or they can do all the breathing for you. They come in many shapes, sizes and abilities to help you breathe. You can simulate this by playing with a close friend (a very close friend). Put a straw into your mouth and start breathing through it. Have your friend put the other end of the straw into their mouth. Then have him take a deep breath and start blowing air into you as you inhale. Play with it by having your friend sometimes blow hard, very soft, fast or slow. Have him blow in when you are trying to exhale and practice how you would deal with this conflict.   In this way you can get an idea of how to relax and work with the machine. If you're inhaling while he's blowing there's no conflict. What if he's pushing harder and faster than you're inhaling? It can be uncomfortable but if you relax and let him push, it won't be a problem. What if he pushes gently, just supporting your own effort to inhale?   It will make it easier for you to inhale whatever volume of air you can take in.

The ventilator is used the same way. It can breathe for you by pushing in a set volume of air, using as much pressure as can be safely given, or it can let you inhale your own volume of air, with a set pressure, or it can do a combination of these things. It can be set to give only so many breaths a minute and let you take additional breaths on your own. The machine can even be set to not give you any breaths but just make it easier for you to take a breath by yourself. This is similar to the way the BIPAP/CPAP machines work.   Technology keeps creating ways for the machine to help you because one way does not work in all situations.

Before you're connected to a ventilator, you'll have a tube, like a big straw, put into your nose or your mouth. This process is called being *intubated*. (You're just gonna love this.) This tube will go down your windpipe (*trachea*), between your *vocal cords*, and into your lungs just above where your windpipe branches off in two directions, one to the left lung and one to the right lung. This way the air goes to both lungs. All of the air will flow in the tube, so none of it will be vibrating your vocal cords; this means *you won't be able to talk*. If you try to talk, your vocal cords will hit the tube, and they may get swollen, so you could be very hoarse or have trouble breathing when the tube comes out.

This tube is called an ET tube, (*endotracheal tube, ETT*). It must be kept in *just the right place* in your windpipe. It can go in too far and end up giving air to only one lung. Or it can be out too far and give air to your stomach instead. You'll have a chest x-ray, right there in bed, after the tube is placed to make sure it's okay. The tube is secured by tape or other hold device wrapped snugly around your head and the tube. The tube will be moved daily from one side of your mouth to the other, even to the center, so you won't get sores. You may also have a bite block so that you can't bite the tube and block the airflow.

Because the tube must stay in just the right place it is critical that you do not move it, so your hands may be tied down, you may be sedated, or both. It's very easy when you're sleeping to reach up to scratch your nose and accidentally pull out the tube. Some people deliberately try to remove the tube (can't imagine why), but pulling out the tube can be life threatening, so we'll do all we can to prevent that. We do not want to have to tie your hands. Critical care units are very strict about tying down the patient's hands and have protocols to follow. The bottom line is, we are trying to save your life and, if you can help us by staying calm and not pulling on the tube, all will be so much better. Some people, *not many*, can cope well with this. They do not need drugs nor to be restrained. They can hold the tube stable when being turned, they can touch their face, etc. This is so great. These people tend to get better faster. DUH! This is another reason why being able to cope is so important. Truly, I have to say, I am not sure I could cope that well!

You're used to sucking in air, but remember that the machine may be pushing it in. This is hard for some patients to get used to. You need to be passive and *allow* the machine to push in the air, and you need to get into synch with the breathing pattern it's giving you. If you don't, you could create too much resistance to the machine's pushing, and it will dump the air into the room instead of into your lungs. We will limit how much pressure the machine can use in order to prevent it from "popping" your lungs. This used to be a very common issue with sick lungs. But technological changes have helped.

Spit may pool in your mouth, and you may drool until you learn how to swallow with the tube in place. You'll receive frequent oral care, including having the spit suctioned from your mouth the same way your dentist does.

The spit that comes from your lungs is called *sputum.* One benefit of being intubated is that it allows us to help manage the sputum from your lungs. The sputum from your lungs needs to be coughed out through the tube and removed or you will suck it back into your lungs. So, we'll stick an even smaller tube, called a *suction catheter*, into the ET tube and into the top part of your lungs to make you cough so we can suck out the sputum. Be aware that this will also suck out your air, but you'll get extra oxygen to help you recover. Sometimes, if the spit is too thick we may have to put fluid into your lungs. We try not to do this, but, sometimes you need it.

Suctioning and coughing will take your breath away, make your breathing get out of synch and it can cause you to panic. The more you panic, the harder it'll be to get your breath back. I tell people it is like when you are swimming and inhale water, or, if you are eating/drinking something and you start coughing, you have to control your response so that you don't get worse. You KNOW that you have to get calm, get control and cope with the coughing so that you can get your breath back and not drown. With the machine YOU CAN BE ASSURED you are not going to drown and *will* get your breath back, plus, we will be giving you 100% oxygen to help! You'll get your breath back, and it'll be easier to breathe after the coughing

Sometimes, after all of this, you may get a tickle in your chest that makes you want to cough. This is the same as what you experience at home when you've had a hacking cough. You know it's just irritation and will keep you awake all night with coughing so you try to ignore it and get over it. Same thing here.

If you are the visitor don't be afraid when the alarm goes off every time your loved one coughs. It's supposed to. A better thing is to just say, "Oh honey, that's a great cough." Remind him that we want to get the spit out, that we want him to expand his lungs with a good cough. Then remind him to try to relax, get back in control, and let the machine give him air. If he needs suctioning, call the nurse.

So here you, the patient are: tied down, unable to talk, being drowned and suffocated and the whole time we will be demanding that you stay calm. (Yeah, right!) Coping with this can be very challenging, yet you must, or you will not be ventilated properly. You must think of the ventilator as your *personal tool for breathing*. It is your friend while you are in need. If it's too hard for you to cope or there is too much resistance to the machines pushing in air, you'll be given tranquilizing drugs to help you cope. If necessary, you'll be given doses large enough to make you sleep. The problem with most of these drugs is their amnesic effect; when you start to wake up you don't remember what's going on, so you freak out, receive more drugs, wake up, and freak out again. On and on the cycle keeps repeating itself.

That's why if you're the visitor it's so important that every time you see your loved one wake up, you *reorient him*. You say, "Hey sweetie, you're at Community Hospital in Santa Rosa. You're in the Critical Care Unit. Today is Friday, February 12, 2013 and it's 2:00pm. You've been sick but you're getting better. You have a tube in your mouth that's hooked up to a machine. The machine is helping you breathe. You have to totally relax and let it. You can do it!" If he coughs, remember to tell him what a good cough that was. He may be scared, angry, disoriented and drugged. Don't freak out yourself, just keep reorienting him. You may have to set limits with him, if he wants you to take out his tube. You have to tell him the nurses won't let you and that if he can't settle down the nurse will make you leave. The whole time you should gently be stroking and reassuring him, sending him love. If he's able to stay awake enough, tell him exactly what is going on, why he is there. I don't think it's a good idea to lie or withhold information from patients. They usually know when you do this, and it really decreases their trust. Most people want to know what's going on even if it scares them. I have met very few people who would rather not know. Most important is that you, the visitor, are not freaking out. If it's too hard for you, just leave. Don't wait for his permission. Let the nurse take care of him. (see Part 2 of this book for coping suggestions)

Sometimes, a person's basic personality or life experiences prevent them from coping at all. This causes even more problems in a person with very sick lungs, because even the slightest resistance can prevent ventilation. They need a lot of medicine to keep them asleep. Sometimes they need so much medicine it drops their blood pressure and urine output. Then we need to treat that issue with pressors to increase the blood pressure, etc. Sometimes they need medicine to temporarily paralyze them to stop all resistance. Eventually, if the lungs get better so this person could be off the life support, he'll still need to wake up enough to pass tests that will demonstrate his ability to breathe well enough without it.

When the lungs are well enough, you'll go through a *weaning process*, receiving less and less help from the machine. You'll also receive less and less medicine to keep you sleepy, until you eventually awaken and are aware of the whole experience. If you haven't learned to cope with the ventilator and are still fighting it, you may fail weaning. You will be re-sedated. Again. You can see how important it is for you to cope.

Sometimes when a patient just cannot cope with weaning at al,l we are forced to take a chance. At those times, despite the risk, they may be extubated and, hopefully, they'll do okay when the initial fear of being tied down and unable to talk passes.

If the tube is taken out before your lungs are ready, it may have to be put back in. And if it does have to be put back in, it may be more difficult because of the swelling of your vocal cords from the last tube. It might be impossible to put in and if another airway cannot be made, you could die. That's why your breathing tube won't be removed until you *demonstrate* that you'll be able to breathe without it. If you're doing okay with your weaning, you'll be required to do some little tests to show how strong your ability is to breathe in and out. It's important for us to know that you have the *strength to breathe and to cough out your spit.* If you do, you'll have the tube removed (extubated) and be given oxygen by mask or nasal cannula.

Sometimes, even if you pass the tests, and you're extubated, you may find that it becomes harder and harder to breathe because your lungs are pooping out. They're still not ready to do the "work of breathing" by themselves. In that case you may have to have the tube put back in. And we can try to extubate again another day. Sometimes it is not that your lungs are having problems, but, it is that your vocal chords are too swollen to easily allow air to pass. This can be a life threatening situation.

Some people may have difficulty coming off of the tube/machine and will need to do it slowly over time, perhaps taking several weeks or more. People who need this tube for longer than about seven to ten days will need to have a *tracheostomy.* That is where a little hole is put in your neck and windpipe. Then a short tube similar to an ET tube is put through the hole and into your windpipe. This short tube is called a

Tracheostomy tube (*Trach tube).* This hole is below your vocal cords so they are saved from getting sores or paralysis from long-term use of the ET tube. You can even, eventually, have a special kind of trach tube that allows you to talk. It's wonderful to be able to talk. This tracheostomy can be temporary or permanent.

People who need long term weaning from the ventilator can go to hospitals that specialize in this. They'll receive rehabilitation and strengthening exercises. They can even walk on treadmills while on the ventilator. The whole point is to build up their general health and strength so they can be taken off of the ventilator. Those who need to stay on the ventilator for the rest of their lives use special home ventilators. This is long- term life support.

There are many reasons why a person needs to be intubated and on a ventilator. One of them is when your lungs have a serious reaction and become severely ill. This is called Adult Respiratory Distress Syndrome.

ARDS- Adult Respiratory Distress Syndrome

ARDS is a syndrome that is a result of direct or indirect injury to the lungs. There are many causes, including stress, pneumonia, infections in your body, trauma--too many things to list. ARDS is severe and life threatening; in the past it was always fatal. Although it can still be fatal, with today's better drugs and technology to help support your body you may be able to recover.

In normal lungs the tissue is nice and stretchy and can expand like a balloon when you inhale air. In ARDS the lungs get stiff because there is an inflammatory reaction in the tissues, which fills them up with fluid, protein, white blood cells, etc. Just imagine that your lungs were made of something that doesn't expand, like water soaked thick cardboard. It would be difficult, probably impossible, to inhale. It would even be difficult to push air in. If you push too hard you may pop the lungs, and then you'll need a *chest tube* to re-expand them (See chest tubes). Technology has come a long way in providing new ways for the ventilator to provide your lungs with air, but even still, we will probably need to decrease your body's resistance to having the air pushed in, so you'll be given drugs to keep you asleep and possibly even temporarily paralyzed in order to eliminate any resistance to breathing. Even with all of this it may not be possible to ventilate you. ARDS takes a longer time to heal so it is generally a longer term situation and you may need to switch out your ET Tube and have a tracheostomy tube placed temporarily. It can be a challenging time for you and for us and we will need to work together to help support your body while it tries to heal.

Chest Tubes

Normally the tissue on the outside of your lung is smack dab against the tissue on the inside of your chest, kind of like the skin on salami. This means there is no space there.

Sometimes due to an accident, an infection, after chest surgery, or your lungs pop due to some other problem, you can get air or fluid in that space between the outside of your lung and the inside of your chest. This will then press on your lung. It doesn't take much air or fluid to cause a problem with your breathing. Sometimes, it can be life threatening and is a "Code" situation.

We may put a tube into that artificial space and suction it out. These tubes are put into the side of your chest. Same thing, if you need it for surgery in your chest. However if you need it for a standard "open-heart" surgery, the tubes will be in the front of your chest. Very often you'll feel these tubes as you breathe especially the ones that come out of the front of your chest. Most people say the tubes hurt, so they don't cough and deep breath as well as they should. Remember to use your pain medicine so you can cough and deep breathe regularly, or you'll get sicker.

The tubes will be hooked to a container on the floor or hanging on the side of the bed. They have a suction device in them to pull the unwanted air and fluid out of your chest. Some of the suction devices use water and you'll hear it bubbling. This can be either a very peaceful sound or very annoying. Some systems don't have the bubbling. Do not think you cannot get out of bed and go walking around with these tubes, because you can once your lungs are well enough to handle the activity.

Bronchoscopy

Sometimes we need to do a look-see inside of your lungs to help us understand what is going on in them. We may need to do a biopsy, or, to stop bleeding. Very often we just need to clean them and suction out the sputum that is there so your lungs can ventilate better.

We will insert a tube, which has a little camera on the end of it, into your mouth or through the ET tube and then down into your lungs.

When we do this procedure, we will give you medicine to help with your comfort and anxiety. You won't be put to actual sleep, but, you will not likely remember the procedure. You will be given 100% oxygen.

When it is all done, we will monitor you until you are awake and stable.

SEPSIS

Many times you can get an infection in one part of your body such as your lungs or a sore on your foot and the infection stays there. It stays *local* to the part that is infected. But, sometimes, when the body is fighting an infection, the chemicals that are released into the blood stream to do the fighting, trigger an inflammatory process throughout the whole body. This is Sepsis and can easily progress to Septic Shock which causes severe low blood pressure and decrease circulation of blood, nutrition and waste products to and from your organs. If your organs cannot get fed right and also get rid of waste products they will start to fail. It is a very critical, life threatening situation. You will most likely need one or more drugs called *pressors* to help raise your blood pressure so blood can continue to circulate and feed your organs. Although these pressors are "code- type" drugs they are often still used even if you are a "No Code" because doctors do not always equate Sepsis with "Code- type resuscitation", although it is a slippery slope and can quickly become that. Some patients do not want us to try to stop their bodies from dying and may see this Septic Shock as a "window of opportunity" to have a peaceful passing. If you do feel this way you need to make it clear on your paper work that you do not want pressors in any situation.

Sepsis and Septic Shock can cause injury to multiple organs in your body causing multisystem organ failure.

MULTISYSTEM ORGAN FAILURE –MSOF

You may start out with one organ system in your body being sick such as having pneumonia or a heart attack. But, sometimes the sick organ causes such a *strain* on the other organs in your body that they get sick too. Or, it may be that you have an over-whelming total body reaction to an infection such as in Sepsis and get Septic Shock (see previous section) which can affect the whole body.

When more than one organ in your body is sick it is called *multi-system organ failure*. It is a very serious issue and has a high fatality rate.

Let's say you had a stroke which is an injury the neurological system. Let's say your ability to swallow safely is malfunctioning and you inhale saliva or food into your lungs and get pneumonia. That is two organ systems. Then your pneumonia gets worse and you get septic which in turn decreases the blood pressure. Now you are in shock. This is a third organ system. Now your whole body is not getting enough blood circulation. Your kidneys are being hurt by the low blood and oxygen circulation. That is a fourth organ. They stop making urine which then allows toxins to build up in your body and affects other organs including your brain. This is a very real and all too common example of multiple organs being ill and injured like a domino effect. The risk of death increases with each additional organ system involved. Three systems or more, ill at the same time, tends to be fatal.

KIDNEY

Dialysis

Your kidneys are great recycling and detox plants. When they're not working, either temporarily or permanently, you'll build up fluid and toxins in your body that can send you into a coma and kill you. If your kidneys aren't working well, you need to be connected, intermittently or continuously, to a machine that can filter your blood and/or remove fluid. This is called dialysis.

There are different types of machines and ways for your blood to be filtered   depending upon what type of help your kidneys and blood need and how fast it's being done. When you need your blood filtered for toxins and fluid because your kidneys aren't able to do it this is called Hemodialysis.

Sometimes you don't need your blood filtered; rather, you just need fluid taken off quicker than your kidneys can do it. There are several ways to do this and they have several different names, but for your personal experience it will all seem similar to the Hemodialysis.

There are also some diseases that might respond to filtering the blood for white blood cells or maybe the plasma needs to be exchanged, for example in Myasthenia Gravis and Guillain-Barre.

The above procedures may be daily, or intermittent such as three times a week, sometimes they are 24/7 depending upon what is being treated.

For temporary dialysis in the ICU you'll need a central IV catheter. One type of catheter is called a Quinton Catheter. This is placed in your groin or neck areas. You may be limited in how much you can move around. You'll need to work with your nurse to make sure you are comfortable.

For long-term hemodialysis you'll undergo a surgical procedure to create a connection (*fistula*) between the artery and vein in your arm. This connection is under the skin and can be repeatedly accessed with a needle that will allow you to be hooked up to the kidney machine. People usually go in to a clinic for dialysis three times a week. Hemodialysis is a long-term life support. Eventually you may be able to receive a transplant.

GI TRACT - GASTROINTESTINAL SYSTEM

Your GI tract contains all of the organs from your mouth to your butt. Its primary job is to break down what you put into your mouth, transform it into a fuel your cells can use, and to get rid of the waste your body creates. There are secondary jobs, such as detoxification, the production of insulin, and the elements that make your blood clot so you don't bleed to death, etc. There are a lot of things that can go wrong with the various organs of your GI Tract i.e. ulcers, tumors, bleeding, pancreatitis, liver failure, decreased circulation to, or a rupture of your intestines, gallstones. If any of these become severe, they can make you sick enough to need the various life supports we have discussed. You may even need a liver or pancreas transplant.

In critical care it's normal to give you medicine to prevent stress ulcers.

Esophagogastroduodenoscopy (EGD)

This test is very similar to the Bronchoscopy. It is done to look inside of your stomach and the upper part of the small intestine. It may be done just to see how the tissues are looking or it may be done so we can do procedures to stop bleeding, do a biopsy, etc.

This tube will be inserted into your mouth and down into your stomach, eventually moving into the small intestine. You can actually help guide the tube by swallowing when the doctor asks you to.

You will be given medicine for your comfort and anxiety and just as with the Bronchoscopy you probably will not remember the procedure.

Colonoscopy

This procedure is to done to look at the condition of your Colon. A tube with a camera on the end will be inserted into your anus and moved up inside your large intestine. We can just be checking out your tissues, or may snip off some growths called polyps, do a biopsy, treat you for bleeding, etc.

In order to do most of these things we will need your bowels to be clean so, if you are at home you will stop eating regular food and just take in clear liquids a couple of days prior to the test. Then the night before the test you will have to stop everything but water and will be given bowel cleaning fluid that you need to drink over a couple of hours. It will make you poop, hopefully, until your poop is clear. In the ICU the prep can be done faster, but we still need the clear bowel in order to see.

As with the EGD or Bronchoscopy, you will be given medicine for your comfort and anxiety and you probably will not remember most of the procedure, but, you will not forget the prepping for it and the joy of eating your meal after it!

NGT/OGT/Feeding Tube

The NG tube (nasogastric) or OG tube (oral gastric) is used to either keep your stomach empty, to give you medicines, and/or to feed you liquid nutrition. The hardest aspect of having this tube is the insertion of it. It may also irritate your throat and possibly your sinuses, and that can cause a postnasal drip.

The tube is put into your nose (NG) or through your mouth (OG) and slid down your throat and into the stomach. One problem is that no matter how big you might think your nose is, it might have only a small or crooked turn space inside, so a little force may be needed to push through the turn toward your throat. It can hurt, even bleed. However, we *will* try to do this as gently as possible and can even use numbing gel to help; feel free to ask for the numbing gel. Once the tube gets to the back of your mouth your help is needed, if you can give it, because at this point the tube can either go into your stomach or your lungs. You may be asked to take a sip of water, hold it in your mouth, and then, on the count of three, swallow while at the same time the tube is pushed in. In this way *you can help guide* the tube to the right place. With this tube your stomach fluid (*bile*) can be sucked out. It may seem strange to see the bile coming out of your nose.

If a tube will be used solely to feed you, the NG tube may be removed, and a smaller feeding tube inserted in the same way, but it will go into your stomach and then on into your small intestine. It's a softer tube and easier to handle. You can be fed this way with less risk of vomiting and inhaling the food; however, with this tube we can't empty your stomach if we need to. If a tube is feeding you, you may see it hooked up to a bag or bottle of some milky like fluid.

To see how well you're absorbing this food, we'll use a syringe to pull out the fluid from your stomach and measure the amount. Patients and families can understand this process and watch it with calm and interest. What really freaks them is when we put all of that gooky mess back into the stomach. Well, hey, just close your eyes. That stuff is filled with things that you don't want to lose.

If you need to be fed through a tube for a longer time, or even forever, we will put a little hole into the outside of your belly and insert a tube into your stomach that way. This way you won't get sores in your nose and airway.

Peeing and Pooping

While you are in critical care everything you take into your body and everything you put out will be measured. That includes pee and poop. Whether you're allowed out of bed to use a bathroom or not, your output will still be measured and/or tested. There may not even be a bathroom for you to use. In that case, if you are able to be out of bed, you can use a bedside commode, a Potty-chair. If you have to stay in bed you'll be using a bedpan or urinal.

Commonly though, you'll have a *Foley catheter* to take the urine out of your bladder. This tube is inserted into your urethra, or pee hole, and up into your bladder. The urine then comes out automatically. I won't lie to you, putting this in can be uncomfortable, especially for men with prostrate problems. After the tube is in, it can be annoying and make you feel like you have to pee all of the time. Usually you'll get used to it after several hours or so and that is good because in the critical care unit your urine output is usually measured every hour. It's often very important to know how much fluid your kidneys are putting out. The amount, color, consistency, and odor of your urine can give a lot of information.

When you have to poop, you'll use the bedpan. If you are having a lot of diarrhea, we may insert a rectal tube. Or we might "glue" a bag onto your butt that collects the diarrhea. Part of the reason for doing this is to protect your skin, which can quickly get a painful rash. The skin may even tear and get sores. Believe me, you're not gonna want that.

We'll try to prevent this by using these tubes, bags, and skin creams.

Of course no matter what you are using, we'll clean your bottom for you. It's embarrassing for most people, but this is part of our job; you pay us big bucks to take care of you.

How your poop looks can tell a lot about how you are doing. There are all kinds of poop; it can be yellow, green, brown, red, and black. It can be watery, mushy, jelly like, greasy, soft, or hard. It can smell normal, bloody, or extremely foul, which may indicate a bacterial infection.

Disgusting as this sounds, your spit, pee, and poop, can tell us a lot, so, just remember that we learn a lot about your condition by checking this stuff. It's a lot easier to joke about it than to take it too seriously. Hey, *you* might even have to check out your spit, pee, and poop. So be prepared.

Our mothers taught us to not pee or poop in bed. Nearly comatose patients, or those patients that you can't get to even move, will try to jump out of bed, over the side rails, so they can get to the bathroom. Confused patients can be downright combative because they have to go to the bathroom, and they will not do it in bed. We may have to restrain these patients so they won't hurt themselves. If available we may need a family member to stay with the patient or we may have to have a sitter stay with them. Dealing with them can be challenging because not only can they hurt themselves or the nurses, they get themselves all worked up and have more trouble with their breathing, their heart, or their blood pressure. So if you ever wake up in the hospital and find yourself in some sort of fog but have to pee, just do it in the bed. We'll clean you up.

HEAD

Our brains are the master controllers of our bodies. They are our means of recognition and communication. Every smile, word, or gesture needs a command from the brain. The body cannot live without the brain and your body is one great, bio-electro-mechanical machine that supports the well-being of the brain. Think about it. Every system in the body is involved in a communal effort to keep the brain alive. Without a brain there is no need for a body.

The brain can be hurt by trauma, tumor, infection, inflammation, too little oxygen, too little circulation, too many toxins, high blood pressure, low blood pressure, swelling, bleeding, etc. Anything that increases pressure too much in the skull will send you into a coma.

You might need one or more tests to discover the problem. One test is a *CAT* Scan. This is where you're taken to the x-ray department and made to lie down on a table that is then slid into a doughnut shaped machine that takes very fine x-rays of your head. Or you might need an *MRI*, which is similar, but uses magnetic and radio frequency waves to create the pictures. Each test looks at your head in different ways and can see different kinds of problems.

You might need an *angiogram* similar to what was described in the Heart section, except the catheter is going to the arteries in your head and the dye will circulate in your brain.

Trans Cranial Doppler studies use sound waves to check the blood flow in your head and watch for spasms, narrowing, or blockages of your vessels. This is similar to the echocardiogram in the Heart section.

You might need a *Lumbar Puncture* to check for blood, infections, or high pressure in the fluid that surrounds your brain and spinal cord. This fluid is called the *cerebral spinal fluid (CSF)*. For this procedure you lie on your side in a tight fetal position and, after numbing a spot in your low back, the doctor will insert a needle into your spine to check the pressure and take samples of the CSF. You need to keep your head down after this for maybe several days or you may get an intense headache when you stand up. I once told my son to crawl to the bathroom instead of walking and this help him a lot.

You might need an *EEG (electroencephalogram)* which would be similar to checking the rhythm of your heart, except there are a whole lot more wires that are attached to certain spots on your head. The wires are hooked to a machine that picks up electric signals and prints them as waveforms that the doctor can read.

There are also machines that can watch the flow of chemicals in your brain; the chemicals show up as colors on the monitor (*PET Scan*).

If you've had trauma to your head or spinal column, you'll be transported to a trauma hospital that's capable of doing neurosurgery. Your spine will need to be stabilized to prevent or limit any damage that could cause paralysis. If your head's been hurt, it'll be important to find out if you have any bleeding inside and, if you do, to stop it and to remove the clot if needed. **Be aware that if you have a blow of some kind to your head and you lose consciousness but regain it again in a few minutes, you could have a serious bleed (*epidural*) that could be fatal if you don't seek help immediately**. Also be aware that if you have a blow to the head but don't lose consciousness you may still have a bleed. Symptoms may show up right away but it's possible you might not experience a problem until days, even months later because you could have a slow bleed (subdural). This is common in seniors because age has decreased the size of the brain and allows more room in the skull for blood to build up before the pressure causes symptoms.

Pressure Monitors/Drains

The skull is a bony room that holds the brain and it has only so much space for your brain and the fluid circulating in it. If you get too much fluid, because you are bleeding or because there is a blockage to fluid circulating around the brain, then pressure will build inside your head and push on your brain. This will send you into a *coma*. It can even push part of your brain out of one of the little openings of the skull. This is called a *herniation.* It is lethal. A little tube can be put through your skull and into certain spaces of your brain so that the pressure there can be monitored (*Intracranial pressure – ICP*). You'll see numbers and/or waveforms on the monitor. There's also a tube that allows the fluid to be drained if the pressure gets too high (*Ventriculostomy*). You might have one or both of these devices.

A person who needs this equipment is not likely to be aware or understand what is going on. He'll probably be confused or in a coma. When you come to visit someone who is having a problem with high pressure in their brain, be sure to ask your nurse whether it's okay to stimulate the patient by talking to him or touching him. The nurse may be giving him medicine to keep him in a very deep sleep and won't want him to be stimulated in any way.

The same restriction might apply to a person with an *aneurysm* in their brain. An aneurysm is a weak spot in an artery, kind of like a bald spot on a tire that pouches out. It can pop and bleed. It's important to keep the blood pressure down. Always check with the nurse before stimulating your loved one.

At other times, when high pressure isn't a problem, periods of stimulation and periods of relaxation may be promoted. The amount of stimulation to provide is controversial. Some people say the more constructive stimulation you have the quicker you can re-integrate and heal. Others say to limit the amount to prevent over stimulation that could cause confusion and frustration. Talk to your nurse and doctor about what course is best for your loved one's situation.

Stroke – Brain Attack

A stroke is similar to a heart attack in that for some reason there isn't enough blood flowing to the brain cells. This can be due to blockage, spasm, or bleeding. Recently, strokes are being called Brain Attacks in order to increase awareness of the need for immediate treatment just as you would with a heart attack. In fact, similar treatment and procedures are done for stroke and for heart attack. If your stroke can be treated with clot busting medicine, doctors recommend that you receive the medicine within *three* hours from the time the symptoms begin.

Symptoms to be aware of are numbness, weakness, or paralysis on one side of your body. One side of your face may become droopy and doesn't move as well as the other side. Your vision may be doubled, blurred, blinded, or have blank areas. You may have difficulty swallowing and may drool or choke. Your speech may become slurred or garbled; you may not understand the spoken or written words people are trying to communicate to you. Or, you may understand but not be able to say or write the words to communicate what you want to. These symptoms may come and go, or they may come in one blast and stay. Call 911; do not drive yourself in to the hospital. Remember that time equals brain cell life.

Neurological Status

Whenever your *Neuro status* is being assessed the tests we do will depend upon what problem you came in with. Following are a variety of tests you may experience: you may be constantly assailed by questions designed to reveal your ability to comprehend, to speak, and to give the correct response. Questions such as, "What's your name? Where you are? What year is it?" and, "Why are you here?" are basic tests. Sometimes the constant questioning bugs people so much that they deliberately give wrong answers, and the nurses may not know whether the patient is playing or is really confused. Don't play unless you make it very obvious. You could end up receiving a treatment you didn't need.

A light will be shone into your eyes to check your pupil reaction. We'll ask you to squeeze our hands, to give us a "thumbs up", to move your feet back and forth against pressure, and to do other physical tests which demonstrate whether your brain is able to hear, to understand the request, and has the ability to command the body to perform the movement. We may ask you to say words or to identify objects and we may check to see if you can feel hot/cold or sharp/dull sensations when we touch you.

With a head injury a person's ability to participate in some of these tests can wax and wane. Sometimes they will follow commands and other times maybe not. It can be frustrating when your loved one does something you've asked him to do but when you try to show the nurse, he doesn't do it. Don't worry, the same things happen to nurses and doctors. Don't feel disbelieved when you hear the nurse say to the doctor, "The patient's wife *reports* he squeezed her hand, but I haven't seen it happen." The doctor will do the same thing. He will write, "Nurse reports..." It isn't that we don't believe each other; it's just that we can't say that a patient did something unless we see it happen.

When visiting, you'll tend to test your loved one. Please don't overdo it. If they don't respond after your first question, don't keep pushing. It can be very frustrating to the patient, and while they are in Critical Care such frustration can be harmful. Also, you must remember when testing a loved one that sometimes what you think is a conscious response may only be a reflex. When the patient squeezes your hand, ask them to hold it, then let go. Squeezing can be a reflex, just like a baby does when you put your finger into their hand. On the other hand, when the patient lets go, did he do it on purpose or because his reflex just relaxed? The frustrating thing is sometimes they purposefully respond and other times it's just reflex. Don't be discouraged. Asking for a "thumbs up" can be more definitive. There are different levels of coma and the patient may wax and wane in their *level of consciousness*. It's similar to when you sleep at night, sometimes you sleep deeply, and sometimes you sleep *lightly*.

When checking a person's level of consciousness, we are checking for awareness plus the ability of the brain and body to communicate with each other. First we'll try a *verbal stimulus*, like calling his name. If there is no response we'll try *touching or shaking* him. If there is still no response, we'll give a *painful stimulus* like pinching his fingernail, because we want to see if, one, the body felt it and, two, how does it react.

At different levels of coma the body responds to pain in different ways. At the deepest level, the patient *will not respond* to any stimulus, even pain. As he climbs the scale toward consciousness the first reaction will be a reflexive *stiffening straight out and rotating inward* of the arms and legs. Above that level, the reflex is a *bending* at the elbows, as if they were going to hug something, and the legs will bend at the knees. Above this level, the patient will show *generalized* discomfort to the pain but not be able to tell exactly where it is hurting. Above that, the patient will have awareness of where he hurts, *localize* the pain, and, if his arm can move, he will try to push away the painful stimulus. Above that the patient will be conscious. He's no longer in a coma, but he may still be hard to awaken and keep awake. All throughout this climb to recovery, remember, the coma patient will wax and wane in their level of consciousness.

As the patient climbs to awareness he'll be less and less sleepy and more able to stay awake on his own. Don't be embarrassed if your loved one starts behaving in ways he'd normally not do. He may not be normal at this point. He may not have the inhibitions needed to behave in socially acceptable ways. So if you're very straight-laced wife begins swearing like a sailor or spitting at you, don't worry, it should pass.

Now that the patient can talk to us, we can start testing for *orientation*, and we'll ask all of those annoying questions. Upon becoming more alert and oriented, the patient will be tested for his ability to think (*cognitive ability*), including the ability to read, to do math, to perceive, to interpret, and to solve problems. Hopefully, he will reach the same level of ability he had before his illness.

Meanwhile, he may have had damage to his ability to physically move normally. He may need to relearn some or all of the ability to command his body. He may need a lot of rehabilitation. This is a challenging time for the patient, his family, and the rehabilitation team. It can be rewarding or devastating. Some people have found that they have become happier people as a result of the changes in their brains. It's not unlike the movie *Regarding Henry*, with Harrison Ford and Annette Bening.

If you've had spinal cord injury you will have to deal with temporary or permanent paralysis. If the injury is high enough you'll need to be on a ventilator for the rest of your life. You may need some kind of surgery or mechanical device used to keep your spine in proper stable position. Until then you'll be on a special bed (see Beds). Rehabilitation for spinal cord injuries is also very challenging. It too can be devastating, or it can change your life for the better.

There was a beautiful young woman who'd been engaged to a man who drank too much. She left him because of his drinking. When the man quit drinking, she came back. Returning home from the airport they stopped at a friend's house. While there he had a few drinks. The girl was furious and demanded they leave. While driving home the man made an error in judgment and crashed the car. He was not hurt but she lost both of her legs above the knees and was paralyzed from the waist down. You can imagine the devastation this girl experienced. Yet with the help of her healthcare team and her family she found the will to live, made it off of life support and into rehab. From there she called me and cried because, she said, the therapists were so mean; they kept making her get off of her butt and learn how to take care of herself. Eventually, she succeeded in over-coming her pain and loss. I'll never forget seeing her at a nightclub, lifting herself up in her wheelchair and wiggling her body as she danced. She had found new meaning to her life, became involved with the Canine Companions Corporation, and had a ton of plans for the future.

BURNS

If you're in a burn unit, you may have any or all of the previously described equipment and problems. Treatment depends upon how much of your body is burned and what parts are burned. Initially your fluid needs will be a prime issue because the burns leak. You may have burned lungs, difficulty breathing, dehydration, shock, infections, loss of limbs, etc. You may need skin grafts and repeated treatments dealing with the healing of skin. There may be major psychological trauma and self-image issues. Utilize the team of professionals who are there to help you through this. Be aware of delayed stress reactions to the event, and to the challenges of recovery. Management of pain, itching, and prevention of infection are major considerations. A first or second-degree burn will hurt more than the third or degree burn, because third degree burns destroy the nerve endings. Pain is very individual, so it's important to use some kind of system like the previously mentioned Pain Scale to measure the degree of pain and the effectiveness of your treatment, and it's important to communicate this information.

You'll need to watch closely for signs of infection, so be sure to get clear instructions about this and about how to care for your skin's health and flexibility as it heals. Do not ignore the instructions. Infection can severely complicate a burn.

BEDS

In the past people stayed on bed rest for days, even after giving birth. Over time it was discovered that this caused other problems, like decreased circulation and blood clots, decreased ventilation and pneumonia, bedsores and infection, decrease muscle tone and strength, depression, etc.

If you lay around all day, your body starts thinking, "Man, I feel terrible, I must be dying" and so it starts shutting down. But if you get out of bed it thinks, "Man, I feel terrible, but geez, look, he wants me to work, that must mean I'm not dying." And so your body starts to heal faster, if it can. Today, even in the critical care unit, you'll get out of bed as soon as it is safe to do so. You can be up in a chair while you are still on the ventilator, with multiple IVs, lines, chest tubes, etc.

You may start out by having your bed put into a chair-like position. If you can handle that, but are unable to stand and move to a chair, we'll use a special chair that can be laid flat so that you can be slid onto it, and then it's raised so you're sitting. You go back to bed the same way. Eventually you'll be standing and moving to the chair.

During this time you may have an *air mattress* on your bed to protect your skin. You may even have an *airbed*. The bed may be able to *rotate* you from left to right by deflating one side of the mattress to turn your body, then inflating and deflating the other side. It's very good for your lungs and skin. As you get better and can move yourself in bed, you may have a hard time on these special mattresses because you slip and can't get a good grip to move yourself. If you're well enough to move yourself, ask for a regular mattress.

If you've had a spinal cord injury or even when you have a serious lung problem called ARDS you may be put onto a very firm bed (e.g. Roto- rest) that rotates by actually having the whole bed literally tilt side to side while keeping your body straight and in good alignment by using special bolster pads. This bed has trapdoors underneath it, which allow us to clean your back or put you on the bedpan.

If your ARDS is really in bad shape, sometimes it can help to have you lie on your stomach so that different parts of the lungs are getting used. We may do this with a *proning* bed (e.g. Roto-prone). This bed is similar to the Roto-rest in that it can rotate you side to side, but, it also can turn the whole bed so that you are lying on your stomach *and* rotate you side to side while on your stomach. Your body is securely held in place by enclosure devices and you are heavily sedated.

If you are having severe skin issues such as pressure sores you may be on a Clinitron bed which is a sand bed that air is blown into so that you are "floating" on heated sand.

Technology will continue to make more beds to help you get better.

CIRCULATION DEVICES

The muscle action of walking helps pump blood from your legs back to your heart. When you are bedridden or chair bound for more than a day or so your circulation gets sluggish, and you can get blood clots in your legs. (this can happen on long flights also, so move your legs.) These clots can be very serious, even fatal, if they move from your legs through the right side of your heart and into your lungs, where they can become trapped and block your blood flow. This is called *Pulmonary Embolus.*

You may have devices put on your feet or legs which intermittently squeeze you. There are several kinds, but I call them all Squeezers. Their job is to help your circulation and to prevent blood clots in your legs by massaging your feet or legs and increasing blood flow. People either love them or hate them.

You may get an injection, into your belly, of an anticoagulant medicine. These drugs help decrease clotting, too.

If you're visiting and want to rub your loved one's feet and legs, be careful that you don't massage or squeeze the calves because you could dislodge a blood clot. You can lightly touch to put lotion on their legs but don't do the squeezing; instead you can squeeze and massage the fee. It is kind of like acupressure.

CASTS/TRACTION/ DRAINS

If you were in an accident, you might have a cast on one or more parts of your body, even around your belly and chest. It may feel warm at first, and it can feel very confining until you get used to it. If you notice your pain is getting worse, or parts of your body inside the cast or below it are tingling or going numb, be sure you tell your nurse. If at first you were able to move the toes or fingers below the cast and find later in the day that you can't, tell your nurse right away. As your body heals you may feel itchy. Don't stick anything inside your cast that can cut or irritate your skin. Talk to your nurse about ways to deal with this problem.

You may find that your leg, arm, or head is in some kind of traction device, held there by little pins that were put into you; these are connected by ropes to weights. This is to keep your body part in a certain position. Talk to your nurse and doctor about what they are trying to achieve, so you can assist.

For a fracture in the neck area, you may have a traction device called a halo attached to your head. It circles your head and is pinned into your skull, and it has legs that go down to a vest that you wear. This will force you to move your upper body and head as one unit in order to protect your neck and prevent paralysis. If you're allowed to go home you'll wear this device until your neck heals.

If you've had surgery, you may have one or more drains that pull fluid from your wounds to help them heal. These drains may be self-contained little round balls or similar devices that create their own suction, or they may hook to a suction device in the wall. You could have tubes that just drain into your bandages. Drains don't necessarily hurt, but you must be careful to not pull them out.

Afterword

By now you should have enough information to help guide you in making decisions that truly reflect your wishes. Remember that as time passes there will be new drugs, equipment, therapies, procedures to consider, but having some basic concepts should still help you.

I hope that you or your loved ones never need most of this information, and if you do, I hope this book will be of great help to you.

As long as I am around, I am available for you to talk with. You can currently contact me at: imlindai41@gmail.com
www.lindaingalls.com

In Love,
Linda

About the author

Linda Ingalls RN CCRN became and RN in 1975 and began ICU in 1981. In addition to providing care as an ICU nurse, she has experience in the following: mental health nursing, life coaching, consulting, teaching, Healing Touch, and is a graduate of the Berkeley Psychic Institute. Linda has received several nursing awards.

She is passionate about informing and empowering people to make choices based upon Love not fear.